Pushing for Midwives

Christa Craven

Pushing for Midwives

*Homebirth Mothers and the
Reproductive Rights Movement*

TEMPLE UNIVERSITY PRESS
Philadelphia

Christa Craven is an Assistant Professor of Anthropology and Women's, Gender, and Sexuality Studies at the College of Wooster.

TEMPLE UNIVERSITY PRESS
Philadelphia, Pennsylvania 19122
www.temple.edu/tempress

Copyright © 2010 by Temple University
All rights reserved
Published 2010

Library of Congress Cataloging-in-Publication Data

Craven, Christa.
   Pushing for midwives : homebirth mothers and the reproductive
rights movement / Christa Craven.
      p. cm.
   Includes bibliographical references.
   ISBN 978-1-4399-0219-6 (hardcover : alk. paper) — ISBN 978-1-4399-0220-2
(pbk. : alk. paper) — ISBN 978-1-4399-0221-9 (e-book)   1. Midwifery.
2. Reproductive rights.   3. Midwifery—Virginia.   4. Reproductive
rights—Virginia.   I. Title.
   RG950.C73 2011
   618.2—dc22

                                                        2010008811

♾ The paper used in this publication meets the requirements of the
American National Standard for Information Sciences—Permanence
of Paper for Printed Library Materials, ANSI Z39.48-1992

Printed in the United States of America

2 4 6 8 9 7 5 3 1

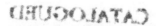

Contents

Acknowledgments   vii

Notes on Research and Activism   ix

Introduction: Pushing for Midwives   1

1 Histories of Struggle   24

2 The Birth of Consumer Activism for Midwives   40

3 Midwives in Virginia   61

4 Mothers in the Legislature   79

5 "I'm Not Really Politically Active, but . . ."   97

6 Divisive Strategies   115

Epilogue: Beyond Consumer Rights   139

Notes   149

Bibliography   181

Index   201

Acknowledgments

I am most deeply indebted to the Virginia midwives and their supporters who so generously gave of their time to talk to me, teach me, and affirm my commitment to a wide range of birth options for all women. Many of you read drafts of my writing, engaged me in thoughtful (and sometimes heated) conversations, sent me hard-to-find articles from your personal archives, included me in wonderful homeschool field trips, and offered me assistance in countless ways. I am particularly grateful to Alice Bailis, Steve Cochran, Juliana Fehr, Ellen Hamblet, Marsha Jackson, Jessica Jordan, Leslie Payne, Brynne Potter, Katie Prown, Patty Ogden, D'Anne Remocaldo, and Lois Smith.

This book would also never have been completed without the support of friends, colleagues, students, and mentors who helped clarify and strengthen my arguments, offered snappy titles, and read version upon version of my writing. During our research support meetings, Mindy Michels and Tricia Silver, and later Jennifer Graber and Amber Garcia, gave me much-needed infusions of wisdom and gently nudged me to stay on task. Writing "boot camp," with Raymond Gunn, Leslie Wingard, Seiko Matsuzawa, and Mazen Naous, provided an inspiring model of collaborative and interdisciplinary scholarly work. My thanks also go to Mary Bader, Tom Boellstorff, Robbie Davis-Floyd, Susan Erikson, Brandy MacDonald, Martin Manalansan, Jeff Maskovsky, Heather McClure, Charles Peterson, Denis Provencher, Heidi Schultz, Thomas Tierney, David Valentine, and Maria Vesperi for their insightful critiques and support along the way. And thank you in particular to Dána-Ain Davis and Mary Gray, whose friendship and intellectual collaboration have consistently reminded me that doing *good* feminist ethnography keeps us passionate about engaging in efforts to advocate for and with those we study. Likewise, I thank my friends and my students for continually renewing my excitement about the power of community-based grassroots activism, especially Deena Fidas, Krissi Jimroglou, Amy Schriefer, Cara Stoddard, and Tom Wolfe. And I am forever grateful to my dissertation committee, William L. Leap, Brett Williams, Susan Virginia Mead, and, unofficially, Sabiyha Prince, who all supported me with their constructive insights as this project began and matured. Of course, all of the above are absolved of any analytical shortcomings or errors in what I have chosen to make of their critical insights.

During various stages of research and writing, I received financial and research support from American University and the College of Wooster. Asan Askin, Janet Gallay, Anna Inazu, Robbie Kaplan, and Emily Tumpson provided kind assistance in the transcription of selected interviews. I also thank Hilary Hicks, Marnie Zoldessy, and Claire Miller, my research assistants at the College of Wooster, for their sharp editorial eyes and attention to detail as they helped me complete the final revisions to this manuscript. Micah Kleit, and his staff at Temple University Press, have also been instrumental to the completion of this book. They not only deftly shepherded my work through the production process, but helped me realize my goal of publishing for a wide variety of readers, including reproductive rights and childbirth activists, as well as scholars concerned with (and committed to) grass roots organizing for midwifery and reproductive justice.

Finally, I cannot thank my family enough for their support as I have engaged in this project over the last ten years: my parents, Donna and Stephen Craven, for supporting me on innumerable and immeasurable levels, David Craven, for offering sorely needed comic relief, Rosalie and Joe Murphy and JoAnn, Brett, Eric, and Áine Waller, for making follow-up fieldwork a joy on both ends, and, most especially, B Murphy, for always believing in me and encouraging my growth as a scholar-activist, a teacher, and now a parent. May I have a lifetime to express my gratitude.

Portions of Chapters 4 and 5 were first published as "Claiming Respectable American Motherhood: Homebirth Mothers, Medical Officials, and the State," *Medical Anthropology Quarterly* 19, no. 2 (2005): 194–215. Portions of Chapters 5 and 6 were first published as "A 'Consumer's Right' to Choose a Midwife: Shifting Meanings for Reproductive Rights under Neoliberalism," *American Anthropologist* 109, no. 4 (2007): 701–712.

Notes on Research and Activism

Social scientists in general have argued for the validity of
midwifery as a socially, culturally, and clinically significant
practice, and have supported its legal and political recognition in Canada and the United States through activism,
writing and teaching. Thus, the relationship between
feminist social science research and midwifery has been
a symbiotic one.
> —Margaret MacDonald and Ivy Lynn Bourgeault,
> "The Politics of Representation"

When I first began working with midwifery supporters in Virginia in 1999, I was already well steeped in the research of scholars studying reproduction who had become activists—including vocal proponents of the natural childbirth movement, such as Margaret Mead and Ashley Montagu, and later supporters of midwives, such as Brigitte Jordan, Sheila Kitzinger, Barbara Katz Rothman, and Robbie Davis-Floyd, among many others. Like many of these authors, I initially struggled with questions about how I would oscillate between my role as a feminist researcher, committed to the rigorous study of reproductive rights activism, and my role as an activist committed to reproductive justice. Ultimately, I followed the activist inclinations of my predecessors who had studied midwives, by conducting research specifically with supporters of midwifery—primarily homebirth mothers. I made this strategic choice in an effort to underscore the importance of women's voices, particularly those women who lacked the resources to mobilize against the powerful (largely male) medical lobby that worked to block legislation to protect midwives. While medical officials' voices were featured prominently in public debate and in published opinions against midwifery, my research sought to raise the volume of the voices of women affected by these policies.

Situating my research as feminist ethnography allowed me to base much of my study in what social scientists describe as "participant-observation," intensive involvement with a group over an extended period of time. As part of this involvement, I frequently joined midwifery supporters in the public advocacy efforts in Virginia between 1999 and 2005. After conducting in-depth interviews with Virginia midwifery advocates in 2001 and 2002, I was asked to serve for one year as a legislative advisor for the Commonwealth Mid-wives Alliance. I continued my service on the executive board of Virginia Friends of Midwives (VFOM) the following year, as I began to write up my research. Upon the completion of my study, I presented portions of it in 2004 to the Virginia Governor's Work Group on Rural Obstetrical Care, with recom-mendations to license certified professional midwives (CPMs) and remove reg-ulations requiring physician supervision for certified nurse-midwives (CNMs). Throughout my fieldwork and writing process, I also presented my research at numerous local and national conferences dedicated to the support of midwifery, including meetings of the Midwives Alliance of North America.

My active involvement in midwifery activism throughout my study also heightened my awareness of another aspect of feminist ethnography that I have long admired: the effort on the part of many feminist researchers to situate their own background, experience, and commitments with reference to those who participate in their research.[1] For me, the value of this endeavor is in demon-strating that feminist ethnography is never an objective enterprise. We all come to our research with our own backgrounds, which allow us—to invoke the words of feminist biologist and philosopher Donna Haraway—our own distinctively "situated knowledges" and uniquely "partial perspectives."[2]

As a white researcher who came from a largely upper-middle-class socio-economic background, it was initially easy to "fit in" with many local and national midwifery organizers, who often shared similar backgrounds.[3] Yet feminist scholarly and activist work has long demonstrated the importance of addressing the diversity of women's experiences—particularly as they relate to race, class, nation, and sexuality.[4] Although midwifery organizers are fre-quently characterized in the media (and sometimes by scholars and activists themselves) as a relatively homogenous group—white, middle-class, North American, married and heterosexual women—I heard significant differences in the experiences and expectations of individual women when I interviewed homebirth mothers in Virginia. The unevenness of their experiences was par-ticularly profound regarding women's encounters with medical officials, legis-lators, and other midwifery supporters, as well as their reasons for seeking midwives.

Thus I found myself troubled by the way some organizers heralded the midwifery movement as a partnership of "sisters in struggle." If we assume that women are all oppressed in similar ways and that "race, class, and sexu-ality only complicate a fundamental gender oppression [it] does not require that relations of domination *between* women be taken into account."[5] In an effort to unite my ardent support of the midwifery movement and my concerns about oversimplifying women's collective and individual efforts to support midwives, I have worked in this book to acknowledge—and at times to highlight—difference in a group that is not always as uniform as it may first appear.

As I became more involved in my fieldwork, areas of difference in my relationship to Virginia's midwifery advocates also surfaced. Although, like many participants, I had been born in Virginia, I had moved away when I was six. My father's job in the U.S. Foreign Service gave my family the opportunity to live and later return "home" to Austria, Germany, Taiwan, and Singapore, as well as Florida, Hawai'i, Maryland, and Washington, D.C. In addition to providing an eclectic upbringing, this experience made Virginia simultaneously familiar and "foreign" soil. Like Lila Abu-Lughod, a Palestinian-American anthropologist who conducted research in the Middle East, I found myself in the peculiar position of being a "halfie," one who conducts research as both an "insider" and an "outsider." Although some have criticized the supposed "easy slide into subjectivity" for researchers who share background or experience with participants in their studies, Abu-Lughod emphasizes how "what we call the outside is [also] a position *within* a larger political-historical complex."[6] Thus I was not surprised when the lines between my insider and outsider status became blurred at various points in my fieldwork.

In fact, it became clear that my insider-outsider status was constantly under negotiation, oftentimes in unexpected and complicated ways. In one instance, for example, an organizer who had been born and raised in New York denied my access to a Listserv to support Virginia midwives because I was not a "Virginia citizen." My decision to rent an apartment in Maryland (about a twenty-minute drive from the Virginia state line) established me firmly as an "outsider." In other situations, I was pleasantly surprised at being considered a kindred spirit in communities where I doubted my ability to fit in. For instance, when I confided to several rural participants that I had insecurities about being too much of a "city girl" when I visited their community during fieldwork, they noted my (admittedly unconscious) decision to leave my car doors unlocked on the first night I stayed with their family. They explained that, for them, this had confirmed my appreciation of "the simple comforts of rural living," including the safety they felt with members of their close-knit rural community. Ironically perhaps, the urban and suburban settings where I met other midwifery supporters frequently proved less familiar than I initially expected. The visible affluence of some participants near metropolitan areas, for instance—from their spacious single-family homes to their designer diaper bags to their commitment to midwives as "the best care money can buy"—differed sharply from my own young life growing up in a duplex and later in a townhouse in the northern Virginia suburbs.

My reproductive history has also positioned me as neither firmly an in-sider nor an outsider with midwifery advocates. Undoubtedly, working with midwives and homebirth mothers has offered me a more tangible vision of what I wanted my own pregnancy, birth, and experience of motherhood to look like and feel like. When I began conducting fieldwork for this project, I had never been pregnant myself. As one homebirth mother reminded me early in my fieldwork, after she spotted me awkwardly cradling a crying new-born during a trip to the Virginia legislature, "Your politics seem to be in the right place, Christa, but we're going to have to teach you a thing or two about what it *really* means to be a homebirth mom." Although I was in my mid-twenties when I began this research, I had known that I wanted children since my childhood, when I used to play "giving birth" with my baby dolls. My mother was a Lamaze instructor and used to borrow my dolls for demonstrations, so I was intimately familiar with the childbirth process, even at an early age.

When I became pregnant in 2009, I had no question about where and with whom I wanted to give birth. My partner and I sought out a homebirth midwife in Ohio, a state where no legislation currently exists regarding mid-wives who are not licensed as nurses and who practice primarily in hospitals. In large part, the decision to find an unlicensed homebirth midwife rested on our experiences and comfort with the skills and expertise of the midwives we had met and worked with in our respective fields—I, as a researcher and an activist for midwives, and she, as a labor and delivery nurse, who had worked with nurse-midwives in the hospital and homebirth midwives after transfers. A second factor involved our current residence in a historically conservative Ohio county. Local residents had been both locally and nationally active in efforts to deny lesbian, gay, bisexual, and transgender (LGBT) people rights to equal access to housing, nondiscrimination in the workplace, and legal recognition through marriage, domestic partnership, or adoption. As a couple who is not legally recognized in our state, we were also drawn to the mid-wifery community's commitment to inclusivity and respect for diverse family structures.

Although in my research I was initially concerned that my relationship with a woman would limit my study to the more progressive homebirthers who also supported LGBT rights, my sexual identity had rarely come up in my discussions with midwifery advocates—either progressive or conserva-tive. Many asked me directly about whether I planned to have children, but I do not recall being questioned about my marital or relationship status—indicating, perhaps, the assumed heterosexuality of those who take an inter-est in childbirth and in midwives. I was "out" to the participants I came to know well, and my relatively "femme" appearance meant that I was not visibly indentified by most participants (as far as I know).[7] On one occasion, when

I discussed my female partner with a participant who I knew came from a conservative background, I was met with an unexpected response. Attesting to the buzz of informal networks of midwifery supporters, she explained that this disclosure came as no surprise, but she was also very honest that she "did not agree with homosexuality." Nonetheless, she made it clear that she did not wish to end what had become for both of us a friendship beyond my fieldwork.[8] Although midwifery supporters have a broad range of political and religious convictions, I was continually struck by the energy that so many midwives and homebirthers devoted to finding commonality around their desire to support midwives—even, and sometimes especially, when faced with worldviews, opinions, and families that differed substantially from their own. This commitment to inclusivity offers a hopeful vision for the future of efforts to mobilize a broad range of families around midwifery. This is particularly important to keep in mind as we consider the tensions I highlight in this book that have emerged around socioeconomic class and racialized identity.

Ultimately, the experience my partner and I had working with a home birth midwife in Ohio mirrored the accolades I had heard from so many homebirth mothers during my research. Our appointments with our midwife frequently lasted upward of two hours; she offered resources on many aspects of childbirth, and she attended to our physical, emotional, legal, and spiritual concerns about the birth process. Yet despite obvious similarities to what I had heard among women in my study, I initially resisted considering my pregnancy and prenatal visits as part of my research for this project. In fact, I actively avoided "theorizing my own experience," as I so often ask my students to do in the classroom. In one instance, after I explained my occupation and research (and my partner's work as a labor and delivery nurse) to our childbirth instructor, she asked, "So, why do you want to take a childbirth education class anyway? Don't you already know all this stuff?" In fact, I *had* attended countless childbirth education classes over the course of my life but mostly in order to study the strategies educators employed and how parents responded. I had never had the occasion to think about the birth of *my own* child. I fumbled around trying to explain this and ultimately blurted out (perhaps desperately) that I just wanted to be a "normal pregnant mom" and to take a class on which I was not conducting any research.

Yet perhaps unavoidably for those of us who engage in reflexive feminist research, my study of homebirth mothers and my personal experience did eventually collide in complex ways when we experienced something every parent dreads. Well into my second trimester, long after we had shared our expectant joy with family and friends, we lost our baby. Mercifully, our midwife continued her expert care for us during this raw and emotional time (and I should hasten to add that she did so for no fee, despite our efforts to compensate her for her time and expertise). Ultimately, I became a "participant-observer" when I least expected it, albeit reluctantly, in my role as a grieving parent. And, despite the painful nature of this time, I count it among the most influential experiences in my fieldwork.

Losing our baby Lily as I completed this project gave me a visceral connection to the two things I have come to value most about midwives: their genuine compassion for women and families in their care, and their versatility in the face of women's different needs during and after their pregnancies. This experience also intimately shaped the way I have approached writing this book—as both a feminist researcher and an activist mother. The care we received from our midwife during this loss, as well as the support we received from other friends who are midwives and the teaching hospital staff of interns, residents, and nurses who cared for us when complications arose, reinforced my commitment to advocate for women's right and ability to access a diverse array of reproductive healthcare options.

Although this book is, in some ways, the written conclusion of a decade of my fieldwork and activism with midwives, I cannot imagine putting this subject down with any kind of finality. There is still far too much work to be done to guarantee women's access to the quality reproductive care they desire and deserve. I believe that supporting women's ability to access midwives and homebirth is central to this feminist vision of reproductive justice. Thus it is my hope that this book will contribute to the continued efforts to expand access to midwives now and for the generations to come. This book is dedicated to Lily's memory and the inspiration she gave me to continue in this struggle.

Pushing for Midwives

Introduction
Pushing for Midwives

Homebirth Mothers and the
Reproductive Rights Movement

Access to professional midwifery care is a basic reproductive
right that women in the United States have long been
denied. Today American midwives are growing in numbers
and in organizational and legal strength. Their excellent
outcomes and women's high levels of satisfaction with their
care are placing increasing pressure on the health care
system to more fully incorporate them, but the battle to
make midwifery care readily available to all women is far
from won. [Certified nurse midwives] around the country
all too often find themselves pushed out of practice by
physicians seeking to eliminate the competition, and
[direct-entry midwives] are still fighting in many states for
the right to practice legally and under regulations that do
not erode their autonomy. It is to be hoped that . . .
American women will be able to reclaim their basic
reproductive right to midwifery care.
> —DEBORAH CORDERO FIEDLER AND ROBBIE DAVIS-FLOYD,
> "MIDWIFERY AS A REPRODUCTIVE RIGHT"

In 2008, the Big Push for Midwives launched a nationally coordinated campaign to gain legal access to certified professional midwives (CPMs), a national certification for direct-entry midwives (DEMs) who are independent
birthcare practitioners and the primary attendants of homebirth in the United
States.[1] Organized primarily by homebirth mothers, the Big Push advocates
"women['s] right to choose their maternity care providers and birth settings."[2]
A second national effort aimed at gaining federal recognition of CPMs was
spearheaded in 2009 by the Midwives and Mothers in Action (MAMA) Campaign, a collaborative effort by several professional organizations for midwives
and "consumer" groups supporting midwives.[3] Both of these campaigns have

drawn nationwide public attention to the recent efforts aimed at expanding women's reproductive rights to include access to midwifery care.

This intensified "push" is the continuation of growing support for access to midwives across the nation since the 1970s that has paralleled (but in some cases been at odds with) the broader reproductive rights movement. Many midwifery supporters have initially been hesitant to describe their struggle as one for reproductive rights because of associations with feminist efforts for women's choice regarding abortion and contraception. Yet midwifery organizers—including those who identify as pro-choice *and* pro-life—have adopted the language of "rights" and "choice" to describe the importance of expanding women's maternity care options. Recent scholarly and popular books have described midwifery as "a global feminist issue"[4] and have positioned the right to birth where and with whom one chooses as a "basic reproductive right."[5] Over the past decade, organizers have also begun to cast access to midwifery as a "consumer rights" issue—one in which a woman's "right to choose" has been restricted by ill-informed public policies concerning midwives and homebirth. Although, as of this writing in 2010, DEMs are legally authorized to practice in approximately half of the United States—owing largely to the successful state-by-state grassroots organizing efforts of homebirth mothers to legalize their practice—struggles for access to midwives continue throughout the country.[6]

It was as this movement was gaining steam in the late 1990s that I began to study and participate in efforts to increase access to midwives in Virginia—where performing midwifery services had been restricted to certified nurse-midwives (CNMs), and those who had been previously permitted, since 1976.[7] Although some CNMs offer homebirth and birth center care in Virginia, since they require "physician supervision" to practice, most currently practice in hospitals.[8] Beginning in the 1990s, homebirth mothers and other midwifery supporters worked for eight years to gain access to midwives who would—and could legally—attend their homebirths. They were finally successful when Virginia lawmakers voted to license and regulate nationally recognized CPMs in 2005 and to loosen restrictions on CNMs in 2006. These local victories in Virginia have also proved valuable on the national scene. Many organizers in other states have sought advice and support from Virginia midwives and their supporters as they now embark on efforts to gain legal access to midwives in their own state legislatures and in national efforts for federal recognition of CPMs.[9]

In this historical moment, when the growing demand for midwives is coalescing into successful lobbying efforts to loosen restrictions on their ability to provide homebirths throughout the United States, it is crucial for activists and scholars to reflect on these struggles for "access to midwifery care for all women" (as the Midwives Alliance of North America advocates[10]) in light of the uneven access women have—and have historically had—to reproductive healthcare. Anthropologists Faye Ginsburg and Rayna Rapp have called this differential access to reproductive services "stratified reproduction"—the power relations that empower some women to nurture and reproduce but disempower and constrain others.[11] Using this framework to address struggles for reproductive rights—both historically and presently—it becomes evident that despite the best efforts of activists, reproductive healthcare reforms have not always succeeded in ameliorating uneven access to reproductive technologies and services, even when enhancing access to reproductive options for *all* women has been the stated goal of activist efforts. In this context, it is important for both activists and scholars to ask the following questions: How is the increasing commodification of maternity care in the United States affecting women's efforts to secure access to midwives? Are all women ultimately benefiting from the enhanced market of reproductive services emerging in the twenty-first century, including midwifery services? What are the possibilities and the limitations of the increasingly popular strategy of advocating for women's "consumer rights" to access midwives and, more broadly, reproductive rights?

Feminist scholars have a particularly important role to play in answering these questions. In fact, feminist social scientists in the natural childbirth movement during the 1960s and 1970s were among the first to offer important critiques of medicalized childbirth, and, as religious studies scholar and homebirth mother Pamela Klassen has explained, to encourage "women to challenge the system through exercising their *consumer power* . . . to turn from obstetricians and hospital birth to midwives and homebirth."[12] Yet while "consumer power" often resonates with middle-class and affluent homebirthers, it has been less applicable to the low-income families seeking midwifery care, who frequently have far fewer "choices" in their reproductive healthcare. While many feminist social scientists—including myself—actively support midwives and women's right to homebirth, we must also consider ways in which our rhetoric of consumer choice, particularly in the context of recent political and economic shifts, may have unintended negative consequences for the very women our strategic suggestions have sought to liberate.

Reproductive Rights as "Consumer Rights"

In the 1960s and 1970s, feminists in the women's health movement adopted the familiar slogan "a woman's right to choose" to demand reproductive rights in North America and throughout the world. This push to characterize reproductive healthcare options in terms of choice and rights is important to contextualize. As historian Rickie Solinger has emphasized in her extensive work on reproductive politics in the United States, the rights language and claims to rights that emerged in the 1960s—particularly within the civil rights movement and feminist organizing of the time—fundamentally reshaped both American politics and culture.[13] Reproductive rights and struggles for "choice" became central to both of these movements, albeit not always for the same reasons. First, reproductive rights posed a dual threat to the status quo: access to abortion and contraception challenged male authority over women's reproductive capacity, and the right to be free of coerced sterilization and contraception, which had disproportionately affected women of color and poor women in the United States during the early 1900s, contested eugenic notions of white supremacy.[14] Solinger has argued, however, that the almost exclusive focus on women's "right to choose" that emerged within the feminist movement during this time became problematic for efforts to grant reproductive rights to *all* women, because the idea of choice was "intimately connected to the possession of resources. Many Americans . . . developed faith in the idea that women who exercise choice are supposed to be legitimate consumers, women with money."[15] The assumed access to the marketplace of reproductive options that this push for "choice" implied did not take into account the constraints that have historically and presently restricted the reproductive decisions of poor women and women of color. Although the civil rights movement had also sought legislation to guarantee "consumer choice" for African Americans[16]—who had long been denied access to goods and services or forced to seek them in segregated, often substandard, facilities—for many minority women, feminist struggles for the "right to choose" abortion smacked of the racism in previous population-control strategies that had been used to constrain reproduction for women of color and poor women.

Thus recent efforts spearheaded by women of color have criticized the singular focus of feminist organizing for abortion rights in the 1960s and 1970s and called instead for "reproductive justice." This term has been used instead of (and sometimes in addition to) "reproductive rights" to address access to quality, noncoercive reproductive healthcare for all women, especially as they are constrained by "the nexus of systems of oppression based on gender, race, class, sexuality, ability, age and immigration status."[17] Yet although the "choice paradigm" of reproductive rights activism has received much critical attention in recent years, it has remained central to many feminist organizing efforts into the twenty-first century.[18]

By the 1970s, even organizers in the natural childbirth movement—a movement that prided itself on attracting those who identified as both pro-choice *and* pro-life—had begun to envision nonmedicalized childbirth as an important aspect of women's right to choose. Many adopted the term "consumer" as what they felt was an empowering term and a calculated alternative to paternalistic characterizations of the (female) patient and (male) doctor. As sociologist and longtime midwifery supporter Barbara Katz Rothman explains, "A 'consumer,' believe it or not, was a role with more dignity, more power, than that of 'patient.' . . . In a capitalist system, in a fully consumerist world, consumption and the language of consumers is what comes to hand."[19] Similarly, in a collection of studies entitled *Consuming Motherhood,* the authors vividly demonstrate how motherhood and consumption were thoroughly enmeshed in North American social life by the turn of the twenty-first century.[20] From the decisions that parents must make to have or adopt children to the commodification of maternity and childrearing practices to the commercial relationships between parents and childbirth practitioners, the "consequences of capitalism for motherhood" have become deeply ingrained in women's experience of childbirth and mothering.[21]

In the case of North American midwifery, for example, Robbie Davis-Floyd, who has described herself as an "anthropological activist who supports all sides of this midwifery story,"[22] argues that midwives engage in a form of "qualified commodification," through which they position themselves as valuable healthcare commodities to "sell" midwifery to legislators, nursing and medical societies, and regulatory boards: "Appropriating the notion of women as agentic consumers of maternity care (an image they [women] helped create), midwives have added themselves to the list of birthcare options from which women can now choose."[23] As Davis-Floyd suggests, mothers now frequently rely on their identities as consumers of maternity care in their struggle to convince legislators and medical officials that they should have the right to choose midwifery care.

In a discussion of how scholars should refer to women who seek midwifery care, anthropologist Margaret MacDonald explains further:

> The term "midwifery consumer" is not to be discarded entirely. . . . It implies a certain agency and choice on the part of women having midwifery care that has always been important to midwifery. Indeed, the consumer-based campaign for choices in childbirth was a key factor that fueled midwifery as a social movement over the last several decades. The idea of the midwifery consumer, however, is not simply a result of the self-conscious feminist agenda of woman-centered care and the critique of biomedicine. It also speaks to the political economy of reproduction within the context of late capitalism and demographic transition, specifically, the trend towards having fewer children later in life and the trend towards treating pregnancy and childbirth as valuable experiences.[24]

In fact, many scholars studying midwifery have also begun to identify themselves as "midwifery consumers" in their efforts to document the important role that women who seek midwives play in legislative efforts to support them.[25]

Yet as Klassen found in her study of religion and homebirth, women who live in the capitalist economy of North America accept the idea of maternity care as a commodity only with "considerable ambivalence."[26] Feminist homebirthers in Klassen's study, for example, resisted metaphors of consumption through religious-based criticisms of the "business of birth." Although many homebirth mothers reject the label "feminist" to describe their support of midwives (in contrast to the many feminist scholars studying midwifery), many express similar critiques of the "business of birth" and instead highlight the importance of the strong emotional bonds they have shared with their midwives and the way that hiring an independent midwife can contest the more dominant medicalized consumerism around childbirth.

Thus it becomes clear that midwifery advocates have a complicated relationship to their identity as consumers. For some homebirth mothers, the act of consumption has offered a way to perform "good" American motherhood, despite their unconventional choice of birth outside the hospital. By highlighting the educated choices they make within the market of reproductive healthcare, middle-class homebirthers are able to align themselves with core American values surrounding consumption. Of course, which practices and values constitute respectable motherhood shift over time, but what links activism for midwives to other historical struggles for reproductive healthcare over the past two hundred years is that in each effort organizers have sought to define participants as good American mothers, and this definition has mirrored the other political and economic concerns of the day. Over the course of the twentieth century, consumer identity became increasingly central to American identity, and thus to activist efforts for social change.

Consumer identity has also offered what many minority organizers have seen as a palatable, perhaps even "neutral," identification (as opposed to, say, feminist activism or reproductive rights) to unify religiously and politically diverse women to support legislative efforts. Yet the focus on "consumer rights" is also intensifying the tensions that reproductive rights advocates have felt historically in the United States—between fighting for individual freedoms (such as a woman's "right to choose") and struggling to increase the availability and accessibility of reproductive healthcare services for all women, particularly those who have historically lacked such access in low-income communities.[27] In this way, the focus on consumption and women's ability to function as consumers has become at odds with broader efforts toward reproductive justice. For low-income women, the notion of claiming "consumers' rights" to hire midwives reveals the significance of socioeconomic divisions within contemporary struggles for reproductive rights. To better understand these contemporary rifts, it is useful to begin with a discussion of historical efforts to enhance reproductive healthcare and their effects on inequities among women.

Revisiting the History of Reproductive Healthcare Struggles

Women have figured prominently in social and political debates over reproductive healthcare in the United States since the 1800s, when they joined the struggle to maintain access to female practitioners through the popular health movement. Women have also engaged in debates over access to fertility control (both for and against legal contraception and abortion) since the late 1800s. And female reformers led a variety of efforts aimed at improving maternal and infant health throughout the twentieth century. These historical movements have played an important role in reforming U.S. healthcare policy, particularly through the promotion of legislation to improve reproductive healthcare for women.[28] Yet far from being a unified "megamovement," as some women's health scholars have claimed,[29] these efforts were most often localized in particular areas and among particular groups of women. Thus despite shared concerns about reproductive healthcare and access to it for *all* women among many activists, these reforms frequently had uneven outcomes for different constituencies of women, based on location as well as on racialized and socioeconomic divisions.

For example, women's activism for the Sheppard-Towner Maternal and Infancy Protection Act in 1921, which led to the nation's first social welfare policy that directed public funds toward prenatal programs, was spearheaded in large part by northern, white, middle-class and affluent feminists. This effort was linked to women's rights groups' parallel struggle to secure their right to vote (which was successful in 1920). For these women, the act was a widely celebrated success for its improvements to maternal and infant health services in hospitals. For African American women, however, the act did not alter segregationist policies, which relegated their care to substandard wards and denied them access to medical care altogether in many hospitals. The act also led to increased state scrutiny into the childbirth practices of African American women and poor women of all backgrounds—particularly their use of community-based midwives. This increased surveillance generated policies that largely eliminated African American and immigrant midwives by the mid-1900s. Thus while historical policy shifts have frequently enhanced reproductive options for white, middle-class and affluent women, they have often been less successful for women of color and for poor women.

These decidedly unequal experiences have shaped women's concerns about reproduction in distinctive ways and initiated different—and at times contradictory—strategies in efforts to improve reproductive healthcare. In the case of contemporary midwives in the United States and women's efforts to support them, some scholars have expressed concern about "the almost reflexive link" that both activists and scholars have tended to draw between the struggles of African American midwives in the early 1900s and contemporary efforts to increase access to midwifery services.[30] In such accounts—which depict a history of "sisters in struggle" culminating in the "rebirth," "return," "revival," or "reclamation" of midwives—there is often scant attention to how women from different race and class backgrounds have experienced reproductive healthcare or the effects of activists' efforts to "improve" it.[31] As anthropologist Gertrude Fraser's research on the history of African American midwifery in the South makes clear, struggles for "natural childbirth" in the 1960s and 1970s made midwives available only to "low-risk," educated, primarily white women with insurance or the money to pay for their services out of pocket.[32] In contrast, women of color and poor women in the United States (and increasingly middle-class women without insurance) have continued to struggle for access to quality reproductive healthcare both in and out of the hospital.

This book marks a critical departure from romantic ideas about a seamless history of "sisters in struggle" for women's reproductive rights and access to midwives.[33] Instead, the history presented in the first few chapters of this book takes a new starting point: women's role as reproductive healthcare activists (rather than the well-documented history of midwives during the twentieth century). This allows for an important discussion of the historical divisions that have troubled reproductive healthcare movements in the United States—which have frequently centered on racial and socioeconomic tensions. Just as anthropologist Sandra Morgen has argued, "The legacy of racism [and, I would add, classism] within the reproductive and women's health movements remains, but it is contested and there are other voices. Moreover, predominately white [middle-class] women's health organizations have been challenged to better address the[se] injustices."[34] Indeed, it was the work of women of color, active in the reproductive rights movement during the late 1970s and 1980s, that led to the transformation of feminist efforts beyond a narrowly focused pro-choice campaign to one that encompassed a broader commitment to reproductive freedom.[35] This book aims to amplify and add to these critical voices to encourage further reflection on organizing strategies that are proving detrimental to cross-class organizing efforts in the twenty-first century.

The Current Context:
The "Consumer Rights" Era

Choreographed against this broader history of reproductive healthcare activism, shifts in U.S public policy over the past few decades became central to the discussion of reproductive rights struggles at the turn of the twenty-first century. The ideology behind such policy changes has been called *neoliberalism*, a political philosophy that rests on the idea that shifting away from government responsibility for ensuring personal liberties toward a "free," or unregulated, market will ultimately resolve social inequities. Although scholars have rightly cautioned against the over-application of this term in recent scholarship—as an easy scapegoat to blame for all contemporary social and political ills—I draw on it here as one influential piece of the history that has participated in shaping contemporary activist strategies. Despite its influence, however, it is notable that neoliberalism is not a term familiar to many U.S. activists, and thus it is important to outline here in some detail.[36]

Scholars and political analysts have referred to recent political shifts as *neo*liberalism because they reembrace tenets from "classical liberalism," a political philosophy that dates to the seventeenth century, which stressed personal freedoms and limited government. Neoliberalism pushes liberalism's faith in the "free market" further by stressing the government's role in promoting market-based policies that favor the *privatization* of formerly public resources (by transferring ownership from the government to private companies) and the *deregulation* of economic markets (where governments reduce or remove restrictions on businesses with the intent of raising the level of corporate competitiveness to promote higher productivity and efficiency). Thus the state's role has moved beyond protecting the freedoms of individual citizens to safeguarding the ability of corporate entities to compete within the market. The notion of what freedom means in the context of citizenship has also changed.[37] Although neoliberalism still promises citizens "freedom," it is defined almost entirely by their ability to participate in financial markets.

It is important to make clear, however, that neoliberalism was not initially the political project of liberal Democrats in the United States, as its name might first suggest. In fact, neoliberalism emerged in the 1980s as a *conservative* reaction to the welfare state in order to reduce what Republicans saw as "government handouts." In the 1990s, many Democrats joined Republicans in adopting a more market-based policy perspective to appear more moderate around issues such as welfare reform. Ultimately, neoliberalism's focus on consumerism and the government's role in encouraging "free markets" can be seen in the economic ideologies and government policies implemented by politicians from across the political spectrum.[38] Accordingly, during the 1980s and 1990s and into the twenty-first century, legislators have elected to cut formerly public services and social programs (such as Medicaid and welfare) in favor of privatization and deregulation.

What critics have called the "magic of the market," which has captivated such a broad range of politicians throughout the world over the past few decades, is that proponents of neoliberalism consider the "free," deregulated market to be a neutral, fair, and even "beneficent" way of determining citizens' access to resources.[39] Yet what the "liberalized" market and the celebration of individual consumption have meant in the lives of many citizens is that their access to services has become based on their ability to pay for the resources that are available.[40] Not surprisingly, this outcome has had the most detrimental effects on the poor, including a marked increase in the imprisonment of impoverished people in the past few decades as increased government surveillance and unequal punishments (which have also disproportionately affected people of color) have taken the place of welfare and other social service programs.[41] Particularly relevant to discussions of mothering and reproductive healthcare, the incarceration of women—most of whom are mothers of young children and many of whom are pregnant—has also been on the rise, increasing sevenfold since 1980.[42]

Even more broadly, as social theorist David Harvey reminds us in *A Brief History of Neoliberalism*, this political philosophy has come to predominate *all* of our lives:

> The advocates of the neoliberal way now occupy positions of considerable influence in education (the universities and many "think tanks"), in the media, in corporate boardrooms and financial institutions, in key state institutions (treasury departments, the central banks), and also in those international institutions such as the International Monetary Fund (IMF), the World Bank, and the World Trade Organization (WTO) that regulate global finance and trade. Neoliberalism has, in short, become hegemonic as a mode of discourse. It has pervasive effects on ways of thought to the point where it has become incorporated into the common-sense way many of us interpret, live in, and understand the world.[43]

In this way, it is not surprising that the valorization of consumption within political and economic institutions seeped into the language of reproductive healthcare activists in the late twentieth century. As philosopher and social theorist Michel Foucault reminds us, ideologies that discipline our beliefs and behaviors most effectively not only emerge from the powers above (such

as medical institutions or the government) but are ideologies that we internal-
ize ourselves and begin to expect of—and even police within—others.[44]

Yet neoliberalism cannot be seen as a complete or totalizing process—it
has limits, fractures, and fissures, in part because it has been as much a social
and political process as an economic one.[45] Rather, as anthropologists Catherine Kingfisher and Jeff Maskovsky argue, neoliberalism must be understood
as "a set of cultural meanings and practices related to the constitution of personhood, markets, and the state that are emergent in a contested cultural
field."[46] In midwifery advocacy, the shifting cultural expectations associated
with American motherhood in the twenty-first century and the practice of
adopting a consumer identity to advance political efforts for midwives must be
placed within the complicated racialized and class-stratified history of reproductive healthcare activism and resulting policy shifts. Indeed, the inequities
that these new developments have intensified are not new. In fact, they map
quite neatly onto the race- and class-based divisions in access to (and activism
for) reproductive healthcare that appear throughout U.S. history.

The neoliberal understanding of citizen rights as "consumer rights" has
created a particularly troublesome paradox for contemporary reproductive rights
activists—especially those who envision their struggle as one to guarantee reproductive rights for *all* women. The idea of "choice" that served as a central
ethical framework for feminism in the 1960s and 1970s has become increasingly problematic, as it has merged with the neoliberal promotion of consumer
identity that emerged during the 1980s and 1990s.[47] While contemporary organizers have found that arguing for "consumer rights" frequently plays well
with politicians across the political spectrum, the intensified concern with
consumer rights, as opposed to "women's rights" or "citizen rights," highlights—
often inadvertently—the inequities between middle-class and wealthy homebirthers (who can lobby legislators as educated, savvy "consumers" of reproductive services) and low-income homebirthers (who lack access to many of
the reproductive choices available to their more affluent counterparts). My
interviews with low-income homebirthers indicate that this strategy is ultimately leading to contentious divisions among midwifery supporters. Yet these
disparities have the potential of being overlooked by organizers from largely
middle-class backgrounds who conceive of their efforts to support midwives as
benefiting all women equally. As sociologist Sheryl Nestel has critically ex-
plored in her study of race and midwifery in Canada, however, "unexamined
notions of 'global sisterhood' actually reproduce unequal relations of power
between women."[48]

"Access to Midwifery Care for All Women":
Virginia and Beyond

The legal status of DEMs, who train directly as midwives and specialize in out-of-hospital birth, has fluctuated dramatically from state to state in recent years, in part as a result of successful legislative efforts by midwifery supporters. At the time of publication in 2010, DEMs are legally authorized to practice in twenty-seven states, including Virginia.[49] Although CNMs, who practice primarily in hospitals, have legal status in all fifty states and in the District of Columbia, their practices are often restricted by legislation that requires physician supervision and limits prescriptive authority.

Perhaps because the particular goals and legal concerns of midwives and their supporters vary so widely across North America, no single "official" name has been adopted for this contemporary movement, though its national significance is evident in the emergence of national Listservs, online social networking groups, and organizations, such as the Big Push for Midwives and the MAMA Campaign, devoted to the support of midwives. Although some organizers have characterized these struggles as part of the alternative childbirth movement emerging from the natural childbirth movement of the 1960s and 1970s, the midwifery movement, and the homebirth movement, no single name seems to have stuck. Another complicating factor is that many midwifery supporters do not see themselves, or their participation in support of midwives, as explicitly political (discussed in further detail in Chapter 5). Nevertheless, there is a sense of solidarity among many midwifery supporters in their struggle to secure nationwide healthcare policies that support women's access to midwifery care.

Virginia is a particularly useful starting point for exploring this national effort because of the socioeconomic diversity evident among homebirth mothers who engaged in efforts to legalize DEMs. Although low-income women in other states also seek out homebirth midwives, little has been written about the challenges of unifying socioeconomically diverse women in contemporary efforts to support midwives. In the wake of the neoliberal policy shifts discussed earlier, the socioeconomic diversity of contemporary homebirthers poses new challenges for midwifery organizers, particularly as they struggle to unify women who also come from across the political spectrum and from diverse religious backgrounds.[50]

In Virginia, midwifery organizers began this work in 1999, when they launched a successful campaign for a study of DEMs by Virginia's Joint Commission on Health Care. After lawmakers advised legalizing DEMs who had obtained the certified professional midwife credential, midwifery advocates lobbied for pro-midwifery legislation every year from 1999 to 2005. In 2003, legislators struck down Virginia's 1976 statute prohibiting the practice of mid-wifery by those who were not licensed as nurse-midwives (or who held permits prior to that time). This change meant that DEMs could no longer be charged with the misdemeanor of "practicing midwifery without a license"—though they remained vulnerable to possible felony charges for "practicing medicine without a license" or "practicing nurse-midwifery without a license."

Fortunately, no midwives were charged before lawmakers passed a bill to license nationally recognized CPMs as independent professionals (able to prac-tice without physician supervision) in 2005. Legislation in 2006 also reduced physician supervision requirements for CNMs (but did not altogether remove them, as I discuss further in the Epilogue). After these successes, Virginia served as a model for struggles to support midwives in other states. Thus it is an important time to reflect on not only Virginia's successful legislation but also the effects of organizing strategies that can prove divisive in current and future efforts to draw together women from diverse socioeconomic back-grounds in the support of midwives.

I want to be very clear, however, that my goal in encouraging this reflec-tion is *not* to detract from efforts to support midwives. Throughout my research, I have engaged in struggles to support midwives at every step and identify my-self as a strong advocate of midwives—both politically and personally. Thus I am keenly aware of the difficulty midwifery advocates face when considering ways that current strategies might undermine their own efforts to ensure ac-cess to midwives for all women. As historian of Canadian midwifery Lesley Biggs has written in a similar reflection on this conundrum, "Many midwifery advocates and supporters position themselves as 'progressives' and understand the struggle for midwifery to be part of the larger feminist health agenda, pre-sumed to be beneficial to all women."[51] Although this standpoint understand-ably hampers criticisms that question the practical application of this goal, I hope that this book will encourage scholars of reproductive rights, as well as activists struggling for midwives throughout the United States, to engage in critical dialogue about the possibilities as well as the "costs" of envisioning ac-cess to reproductive options as a competition for consumer rights.

From Ethnography to Interdisciplinary Activist Scholarship

Ethnography, the descriptive study of human groups, has long been touted as the foundation of cultural anthropology.[52] Although my academic training is in anthropology, my introduction to ethnography came amid what some have called an "interdisciplinary phenomenon," where research methods involving extended fieldwork, including in-depth interviewing and participant-observation, had become common throughout the social sciences.[53] Most influential to me were the feminist discussions that emerged from a variety of disciplines during the 1980s and 1990s that began to consider what *feminist* ethnography might look like—as a research method but also as a style of writing and application of research concerned with ending injustices and inequalities for women and other vulnerable groups. As an important caution, sociologist Judith Stacey's influential critique "Can There Be a Feminist Ethnography?" questioned whether "the appearance of greater respect for and equality with research subjects" in feminist ethnography could ultimately mask the potential for deeper forms of exploitation.[54] In a second article published (inadvertently) under the same title as Stacey's, anthropologist Lila Abu-Lughod suggested that feminist ethnographers contribute to research on inequality by critically examining ways in which women from privileged backgrounds often contribute to the oppression of more marginalized women by universalizing and romanticizing a shared "women's experience."[55] This concern is particularly relevant to research on and activism within struggles that draw together diverse groups of women. While the relationship between ethnographer and participants in research is always uneven, this tension is heightened when participants have experiences that differ substantially from one another, and thus in many cases from the ethnographer.

As one possibility for mediating the unavoidably imbalanced nature of fieldwork—where various participants often give much of their time and knowledge for little reward—many feminists have envisioned research as inseparable from feminist practice.[56] It is at this point that feminist ethnography goes beyond the scope of applying particular research methods. As anthropologist Faye Harrison explains:

> Methods are specific procedures, operations, or techniques for identifying and collecting the evidence necessary to answer research questions. In and of themselves, they are not feminist or non-feminist. Therefore, there are no "feminist methods" per se. However, there are "feminist methodologies," because methodologies articulate conceptual, theoretical, and ethical perspectives on the whats, whys and hows of research and the production of knowledge. . . . A feminist methodology clues us in on which combination of methods is likely to be most suitable for meeting the pragmatic and ethical objectives of a feminist research project.[57]

A core value of feminist ethnography is to produce research that is meaningful and useful to participants, often by contributing to efforts to combat the

injustices they face. This goal has emerged alongside similar work in the growing field of activist scholarship. Several recent publications have called for a
more engaged, public, and activist orientation within the social sciences.[58] In
Engaged Observer, for instance, anthropologist Victoria Sanford describes the
importance of making scholarship relevant to the people we study: "Activist
scholarship reminds us all that research is inherently political—even, and
perhaps especially, that scholarship presented under the guise of 'objectivity,'
which is no more than a veiled defense of the status quo."[59]

Like many feminist ethnographers, my public and activist work for midwives has stemmed both from previous personal commitment (for me, to reproductive justice)[60] and from my desire to "give back" to the participants in my
study—for their generosity, with both time and resources—in both a meaningful and a useful way. This was also an expectation among many of those who
granted me interviews. For example, in one small, rural community, I soon realized that each person I interviewed had talked with the participants I had
spoken to earlier. Thus each new interview I conducted allowed them to collectively intensify their questions about the purpose of my research and express
their desire that our interviews result in something "for the greater good . . . so
that all women could get access to midwives," including the largely impoverished families in their community. Since so much of the published research on
midwifery and the written testimonies of homebirthers have focused on middle
class women's experiences, a central part of my feminist ethnographic project
has been to highlight the experiences of low-income women—both in my
scholarly work and in conversations with midwifery supporters.

Yet claiming a politics for one's work while still publishing for a primarily
academic audience has been disturbingly common among progressive aca-
demics.[61] Rather, recently scholars have argued that we must consciously move
our research "off the shelf"[62] by making it both accessible and useful to groups
that can ultimately put our work to use far beyond what we could do as individuals. For those of us who are committed to activist scholarship, burnout is
perilously common because many of the organizations with which we work are
often in dire need of volunteers with research skills. In addition to engaging
(prudently, and sometimes cautiously) in these efforts ourselves, making our
work accessible to activists allows us to more effectively put our research into
service for the organizations, people, communities, and issues we study.[63] It is
my belief, and the intent of this book, that feminist ethnography should speak
to a range of audiences—from scholars concerned with social justice to students
of anthropology and feminist research to reproductive rights activists themselves including midwifery supporters. As anthropologist Charles Hale has written, "Activist scholarship embodies a responsibility for results that these 'allies'
can recognize as their own, value in their own terms, and use as they see fit."[64]

Thus I presented summarized data throughout my research process on Listservs and at gatherings of midwifery supporters to initiate discussions of the limits of "consumer rights" arguments for low-income women. Since many midwives and advocates did not have the time (or necessarily the inclination) to engage with my research on such a deep and involved level—as one organizer explained, "We only ever read one page, Christa, MAX!"—I also had productive conversations about these issues during visits or phone calls with participants, including those who did not have easy access to the Internet. Yet making my research process and analysis so "public" has often also meant entering into difficult conversations—particularly since midwifery supporters are subject to such sustained and unsympathetic critiques by medical officials and oftentimes legislators (as I further outline in Chapter 4). Many midwifery organizers with whom I spoke, particularly at the local and national conferences where I presented my research, saw little reason to question consumer-based language that had proven so useful in conversations with legislators.

While the collaborative strategies I attempted to employ during my fieldwork and writing processes by no means eliminate inequities in the ethnographic encounter (for instance, I ultimately chose the quotes that I include in this book from lengthy transcriptions), my goal has been to mediate the centrality of my own voice and highlight a variety of women's experiences and stories.[65] The collaborative work many midwifery supporters entered into with me during my research—reflecting with me on my initial analyses of interviews and on the themes emerging in legislative testimony,[66] and ultimately assessing my writing at various stages of development—has benefited this book immeasurably, and I am tremendously grateful for their efforts.

The goal of producing scholarship that is accessible—and useful—to a broad range of readers is also particularly challenging for those of us committed to feminist ethnography as a part of interdisciplinary activist scholarship. My research with midwifery supporters, for instance, has taken me on a journey not only through the extensive literature in anthropology and feminist studies on midwives, reproduction, women's activism, and neoliberalism but also through theoretical and empirical scholarship from fields as diverse as American studies, communications, cultural studies, English, ethnic studies, history, philosophy, political science, religious studies, social theory, and sociology. Without intending to absolve myself of appropriate scholarly responsibility, I feel it is important to acknowledge that it is impossible to be an expert in all of these fields. Inevitably, then, my treatment of some sources and theoretical debates is incomplete. Throughout this book, I indicate the disciplinary backgrounds of authors who have influenced my work in order to give the reader a sense of the interdisciplinary—and inherently collaborative—nature of historical and ethnographic inquiries.[67] I also do my best to provide extensive endnotes explaining connections to particular resources in greater detail and referring to additional sources should the reader wish to pursue a topic that is not covered in great depth in my discussion.

Methods for an Activist Ethnography

Despite my visible activism for midwives during my fieldwork, I was attentive to the highly controversial nature of homebirth and midwifery at the turn of the twenty-first century as I sought midwifery supporters to participate in my study. Because many midwives practiced underground when I conducted research in Virginia, I attempted to protect the identities of participants by performing multi-sited research instead of more traditional ethnographic fieldwork conducted in a single community.[68] Since legislative efforts emerged from groups throughout Virginia, and all Virginians would ultimately be governed by statewide legislative decisions, I also considered it important to assess differing reproductive healthcare needs in areas throughout the state.

Thus between 1999 and 2005 I conducted participant-observation with midwives and their supporters at a variety of public events. I attended legislative hearings in Richmond on midwifery laws during each of those years and the judicial proceedings for the trial of a prominent local midwife in 2000. I also joined numerous grassroots organizing meetings of midwifery supporters that occurred in communities throughout the state, with the intent of drawing in homebirthers who could not always travel to other meetings or hearings, and others that were strategically scheduled before or after legislative hearings in Richmond when members from throughout the state came together to support legislation.

After identifying zip codes where the majority of homebirths had been reported in Virginia in 2000,[69] I conducted semi-structured interviews with forty midwifery supporters during 2001 and 2002 in and around Albemarle County (around Charlottesville), Chesterfield County (near Richmond), Fairfax County (in northern Virginia), Floyd County (southwest of Roanoke), Fredrick and Clarke Counties (near Winchester), Louisa County (to the east of Charlottesville), Richmond City, Stafford County (in Central Virginia), and Virginia Beach County (in the Tidewater area). See the Virginia County Map that highlights my research areas.

Because participants frequently introduced me to other homebirthers when I visited their communities, many interviews occurred as a result of snowball sampling (though I met numerous organizers initially at legislative hearings in Richmond). Although interviews frequently took the form of a conversation between the participant and me (and often their children as they played nearby), I asked all participants to discuss (1) their reasons for supporting homebirth

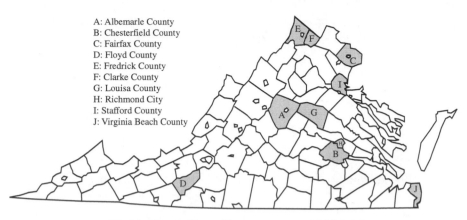

A: Albemarle County
B: Chesterfield County
C: Fairfax County
D: Floyd County
E: Fredrick County
F: Clarke County
G: Louisa County
H: Richmond City
I: Stafford County
J: Virginia Beach County

Virginia County Map with research areas highlighted.

and midwifery; (2) the social, political, and economic barriers to that support; and (3) their expectations about political participation and grassroots organizing.[70] In 2007, I also conducted follow-up interviews with six of the original participants and several new midwives to assess what changes had occurred since the passage of the 2005 legislation that provided licensure for CPMs. Each interview was recorded, transcribed, and analyzed in the context of the public debates over midwifery and homebirth and the several thousand e-mails I collected during my participation on local and national Listservs dedicated to the support of midwifery from 1999 to 2005.

Although most participants were eager to tell their stories about homebirth and their support of midwives, and I have maintained contact with many who became good friends during my fieldwork, others refused interviews with all "reporters," and many participants admitted to "checking around about me" with other homebirthers before agreeing to interviews.[71] Others, citing my prominent involvement with a variety of grassroots organizations to support midwives, initially declined my requests for interviews, suggesting that they would not have anything to offer regarding the "political" struggle for midwifery. Although my dual role as researcher and activist was no doubt a limitation to the study in some cases, many participants also reported that our meetings had prompted them to reconnect with other midwifery supporters, and, for some, to (re)engage in organizing efforts to enhance access to homebirth midwifery services. Others requested updates on the current legislative developments and other grassroots organizing goals. Thus for many homebirthers I became not only a researcher but also a grassroots organizing resource.

Midwifery Supporters in Virginia

In contrast to many ethnographers who "thickly describe" the participants in their studies,[72] I often withhold identifying characteristics of individual participants, given that practicing midwifery (without a nurse-midwifery license) was a criminal offense during much of my fieldwork in Virginia. Despite the limitations I placed on my research questions—with the aim of focusing solely on grassroots organizing for midwifery—many women chose to share their childbirth experiences with me, often including narratives about their deliveries with underground midwives in Virginia. Thus, to protect the identity of the participants, the quotes from the interviews I conducted and the majority of Listserv correspondence I collected for this project are referenced only with pseudonyms and identified only by the year they took place. Quotes that identify a participant's practice as a midwife are referenced as "unnamed participant" to prevent identification of the speaker by quotes included elsewhere. I also made every effort to contact participants quoted in this book to secure their permission to publish the specific statements I chose to include. Accordingly, I respected the wishes of participants who preferred not to risk identification by removing their stories.

On the whole, it has been primarily educated, white women—from a broad range of political and religious backgrounds[73] and from both urban and rural areas of the state[74]—who have sought to enhance access to midwives in Virginia. While participants in my study mirrored national homebirth trends in many ways, they departed from the national statistics on those seeking homebirth as being largely middle class.[75] Although it was not the initial intent of my study to focus on socioeconomic differences among midwifery supporters, it became clear through my participant-observation at grassroots organizing meetings and legislative hearings, as well as through my interviews, that class tensions were impacting organizing efforts for midwives in Virginia.

Assessing socioeconomic class, however, has been a perennial challenge for social scientists. It is particularly difficult for researchers who study families that have chosen what scholars and proponents have called "simple living" or "voluntary downshifting," a trend that paralleled interest in homebirth in the late twentieth century.[76] Indeed, some—though certainly not all—of the participants in my study identified with this movement and indicated that they had grown up with more affluent backgrounds than their current circumstances suggested. Others, however, suggested, to the contrary, that they had grown up in poverty and now lived a largely middle-class lifestyle. Thus in any analysis of differing experiences related to relative wealth and poverty, it is important to remember that socioeconomic class can change over time.

In order to tease apart the complicated ways that socioeconomic status affects women's reproductive decisions and experiences, I offer participants' own narratives as often as I can (without risking anonymity) to explain the circumstances that influenced them individually.

I also took a more systematic approach to the sample as a whole. In each interview, among a list of fifteen other demographic questions about religious background, political affiliation, racial and ethnic background, age, household size, and the like, I asked the participant for an estimate of her or his household's annual income and the educational background and occupations of its members. My analysis of the differences between the experiences of low-income homebirthers and those of middle-class and more affluent homebirthers is based in part on these reports. For instance, the participants in my study reported a broad range of annual incomes, ranging from as low as $6,000 to more than $250,000. Two-thirds of the participants lived in households that fell below the median income levels for their county,[77] and nearly one-quarter lived in households that fell below the federal poverty line,[78] though only two acknowledged receiving federal assistance.

My data on occupation and education complicated the socioeconomic picture of midwifery supporters in Virginia. Participants had frequently worked at a variety of different jobs over their lifetimes (sometimes moving between jobs that required an advanced degree and service-level professions), and the education level of participants in my study was generally quite high: all but five participants had taken at least one college course.[79] Sixteen participants in my study had at least some training as midwives, though only six were currently practicing.[80] Of the thirty-four participants who were not practicing as midwives at the time of my study, approximately three-quarters referred to themselves primarily as "stay-at-home moms," although many of these women also worked outside of the home in occupations including work as childbirth-related specialists, alternative healthcare practitioners, teachers, farmers, migrant fruit harvesters, waitresses, and military personnel. Several participants were students, and almost half were homeschooling their children. Income level had frequently changed over the course of a participant's life, and although the participant's discussions of experiences with reproductive healthcare and support of midwives hovered at times around issues related to income, their stories were frequently punctuated by broader experiences of poverty, power, and access to (and experiences with) medical care. Thus measures such as education level, income, and occupation at the time of my study are admittedly imperfect in terms of assessing socioeconomic divides. Further complicating matters, federal poverty levels do not vary by county (which can be significant in states like Virginia, where median income levels vary by over $50,000 between rural and urban areas of the state),[81] and median income levels by county do not take into account family size.

Social scientists have also shown that analyses of socioeconomic status cannot be separated from discussions of how racialized identity is also infused in experiences of medical access, political power, and poverty.[82] Much like the national midwifery movement, participants in my study were predominately white and of northern European descent. Only four women of color (10 percent of my sample)—including African American and American Indian participants, as well as those who identified as "mixed"—agreed to be interviewed for my study, and they were especially concerned about being vulnerable to state intervention as a result of their choice to give birth at home. Thus although I discuss the historical elimination of African American midwives in depth, I withhold the racial or ethnic backgrounds of participants because women of color would be easily identified within contemporary midwifery organizing in Virginia. Instead I rely on participants' own narratives about their (lack of) reproductive choices and their efforts to support midwives to address how their particular circumstances influenced their experiences.[83]

Overview of the Book

This book has two primary sections, reflecting the dual goal of providing a nuanced history of women's reproductive healthcare activism in the United States and examining contemporary organizing strategies for reproductive rights in an era increasingly driven by political rhetoric which prioritizes "consumer rights." Accordingly, Chapters 1–3 offer a historical discussion of struggles over reproductive healthcare in the United States, and Chapters 4–6 address how women's contemporary legislative efforts for midwives—and reproductive rights—have changed in the wake of neoliberalism. Chapter 1 revisits the history of women's political organizing in the popular health movement in the early 1800s, the fertility control debates of the late 1800s, the struggle for access to pain medication in childbirth during the early 1900s, and efforts to improve maternal and infant healthcare, which culminated in the passage of the Sheppard-Towner Maternal and Infancy Protection Act in 1921. The chapter highlights how, despite vast improvements in reproductive healthcare over the past two hundred years (such as lower mortality rates for both mothers and infants), the public policy shifts sought by women's rights activists have often contributed to the further stratification of healthcare options on the basis of race and class.

Chapter 2 takes a more detailed look at the emergence of consumer activism for midwives and the politics surrounding race and class disparities in the natural childbirth movement, a social movement many cite as the impetus for the "midwifery renaissance."[84] Acknowledging some striking similarities to the uneven effects achieved by earlier reproductive healthcare movements, this chapter reviews examples of birthing reform in several states to highlight the mixed effects that successful efforts to legalize and license midwives have had on the ability of women—particularly poor women and African American women—to gain access to them. This history brings up a crucial question about contemporary advocacy strategies: Will market-based advocacy strategies ultimately lead to policies that make midwives available only to middle-class and affluent "consumers"?

Parallel to this broader national history, Chapter 3 provides a rich local history of midwifery and grassroots organizing among homebirth mothers in Virginia. I review the state's efforts to "educate" and ultimately eliminate African American midwives during the early to mid-1900s, the subsequent criminalization of "lay midwifery," and the "rediscovery" of midwives with the resurgence of interest in homebirth during the 1980s and 1990s in Virginia. Ultimately, several "histories of midwifery" emerge that highlight the racialized and classed rhetoric and prejudices that led to the different political, economic, and social climates for midwives during the twentieth century.

Chapter 4 examines the contemporary legislative debates over midwives in Virginia and how they became, vicariously, about the childbirth choices of homebirth mothers. Medical officials (and often legislators) frequently argued that mothers, particularly those who appeared to be politically active in support of midwives, were not competent to make the choice to have a homebirth and that their mothering choices should be protected and regulated by the state. Many challenged the mothering practices of homebirthers by linking them with women they deemed "pathological"—child abusers, negligent mothers, and drug users—and placing them outside the cadre of "normal" American mothers who acknowledge the "natural" superiority of medical childbirth practices. In response, grassroots organizers for midwives sought to reclaim their status as respectable mothers by highlighting their identity as educated consumers struggling in opposition to a powerful, and highly paid, medical lobby.

Chapter 5 explores midwifery supporters' responses to the damaging stereotypes they faced in the legislature. Throughout my fieldwork, it became increasingly clear that the homebirth mothers involved in these efforts avoided labels such as "political activist" or "grassroots organizer" to describe their support of midwifery. Even though most women denied participating in political activism, yet paradoxically engaged in activities that they described as "political," their reasons for doing so were often quite varied. Middle-class women had begun to redefine themselves as consumers (rather than as citizens or activists) to highlight their economic power in the face of well-paid lobbyists, physicians, and public health officials. While they discussed feeling "empowered" and "energized" by their experiences going to the legislature to support midwives, low-income women were frequently more concerned with the potential of state repercussions both for hiring midwives and for participating in political efforts to support them.

In Chapter 6, I consider how the legislative and organizing experiences of homebirth mothers have intersected with neoliberal political ideology to encourage the promotion of "consumer rights" in efforts to gain access to reproductive healthcare services. I begin with a broad overview of "rights discourse" in the United States and consider how key legal cases have shaped (and to a certain extent have been shaped by) activist strategies for supporting reproductive rights. In the contemporary midwifery movement, efforts to secure access to midwives as a "consumer's right" have allowed some homebirthers to claim respectability as mothers who make educated choices in their consumption of childbirth services, but this focus has also restricted the participation of low-income midwifery supporters who do not have the ability to consume such varied childbirth options. In fact, I document how low-income homebirthers encountered challenges to creating coalitions with more affluent homebirthers when their "choice" to use a midwife was influenced by their experiences of poverty and alienation as well as their desire for a personal, warm, and noninterventionist birth experience.

In the Epilogue, I provide an update on the current state of affairs for midwives in Virginia and consider the future for reproductive rights activism in the wake of neoliberalism. In effect, the meaning of a "right" has changed for all citizens in this new political and economic climate. The state's support of "consumer rights"—instead of the protection of *all* citizens' rights—ultimately forces women to compete for their reproductive choices. It is my hope that this book on the growing push for midwives in this "consumer rights" era will serve as a cautionary tale for reproductive rights advocates more generally. Within the midwifery movement itself, it is intended to encourage critical conversation about both the possibilities and limitations of market-based activist strategies and their effects on access to midwives for *all* women.

1

Histories of Struggle

*Activism for Reproductive Healthcare
since the 1800s*

[Academics have a] tendency to homogenize the history of
reproductive health care so that it comes to have, in a sense,
a creation story and then another with a happy ending as
women rediscover their control over birthing and come to
reassert the 'natural' processes of their bodies against the
unnatural technologies of hospital-centered obstetrics.
  —Gertrude Fraser, "Modern Bodies, Modern Minds"

Although the concept of "reproductive rights" emerged in the context of
feminist and civil rights activism in the 1960s and 1970s, struggles
for access to reproductive healthcare have a much longer and complicated history. Not unlike the more recent activism for reproductive freedom—
including access to midwives—these earlier struggles over healthcare reform,
fertility control, twilight sleep, and the improvement of maternal healthcare
are illustrative examples of the historical impact of stratified reproduction.[1]
Although reproductive medicine has functioned as a key site of social control
over all women's bodies during the past two centuries,[2] the strategies of government and medical surveillance have not been deployed evenly. Power relations that are linked to familiar racialized and socioeconomic hierarchies
have encouraged activism that has allowed some women greater freedom in
their reproductive options but has often simultaneously led to the denial of
those options to others. I explore in this chapter how women's organizing efforts to change healthcare can contest, but not usually fundamentally change,
existing power relationships between women, medicine, and the state.[3] Rather,
women's resistance to dominant state and/or medical power frequently reflects—
and even at times reproduces—the uneven ways social control has been implemented among different groups of women. It is also important to remember
that the impacts of historical inequities in healthcare have inescapably continued to affect the different expectations women have about reproduction today,

as well as how they approach efforts to attain reproductive rights and freedoms into the twenty-first century.

Although a great deal of research in recent years has addressed stratified reproduction through new reproductive technologies—both those that promote and control fertility[4]—little attention has been paid to efforts aimed *against* what anthropologist Robbie Davis-Floyd has critiqued as the "technocratic" model of birth in U.S. hospitals.[5] Efforts to expand women's ability to give birth outside of the hospital also indicate the stratified nature of options available to women when one looks historically at the elimination of African American and immigrant midwives, as well as at the present demographics of those who seek homebirths. Historians and social scientists published numerous critiques of the medicalization of childbirth during the twentieth century and women's subsequent "return" to natural childbirth.[6] These books were important to feminists as "counter-narratives that challenge many of the myths and assumptions underlying the 'official' histories of obstetrics."[7] They frequently emphasized the elimination of (almost entirely female) midwives in the early 1900s during the rise of the (predominately male) obstetrical profession in the United States and suggested that contemporary efforts to license midwives are based in an effort to "reclaim" these practitioners for all women. Yet the history of struggles over reproductive healthcare in the United States reveals as much disparity—particularly regarding the ways race and class impacted women's (and midwives') different experiences of medicalization—as it does such continuity.

While medicalization was clearly a key factor in public health efforts to eliminate midwives during the twentieth century, I argue that taking a different starting point to the history of women's recent struggles to secure access to midwives will offer a richer and more honest portrayal of how women have often fought different—and at times conflicting—battles for what have now become known as "reproductive rights." In their struggles, women's health organizers frequently sought to present themselves to state and medical officials as respectable American mothers to advance their cause. Yet, as I discuss in subsequent chapters on the natural childbirth movement and contemporary organizing for midwives, the values they championed, particularly as they reflected American ideologies surrounding race, class, politics, and religion, also significantly influenced both their activist efforts and their outcomes. By revisiting what Gertrude Fraser described earlier as a misleading "creation story" of women "reclaiming" their reproductive rights, this revised history of women's activism for reproductive healthcare over the past two hundred years will offer a more solid foundation from which to explore the reason contemporary reproductive rights efforts must guard against further dividing women's struggle.

The Popular Health Movement and Women's Efforts toward Healthcare Reform

Women's first organized resistance to medicalization in the United States emerged with the popular health movement during the early 1800s. While the movement did not focus on women's healthcare alone, women were prominent leaders who targeted reproductive healthcare specifically for reform.[8] With its beginnings as a populist movement, the popular health movement attracted many farmers, artisans, and working people who found themselves unable to afford rising medical expenses.[9] For these groups, this movement also reinforced the idea that self-care was an important indicator of American self-reliance and democracy.[10] Fearing that proposed state licensure for "regular" medical physicians would eliminate the practices of other healers, many female "lay" healers (a common term at this time to identify healers who were not professionally trained) and their primarily female followers began to fight against the rise of the "regular" medical system, which was composed, almost exclusively, of men.[11]

Instead, the popular health movement advocated for lay control over healthcare and the protection of "irregular" practitioners—those who did not follow a strictly medical training or protocol, such as botanical healers (i.e., Thomsonians, Native American healers, and herbalists), eclectics, hydrotherapists, Grahamites, Seventh-Day Adventists (such as John Harvey Kellogg), and spiritualists. As social historians Rosalyn Baxandall, Linda Gordon, and Susan Reverby have explained, much early organizing in the popular health movement was among middle-class women and men, primarily because the working class was still a minority in the United States and working-class women were "not well organized and . . . most agitation was local, as was most industry, so that mass coordinated efforts were difficult."[12]

The popular health movement also overlapped and collaborated with several other social movements of the time, including the emerging women's rights movement, the organization of religious and socialist utopian communities, the abolitionist movement, and what women's health scholars Barbara Ehrenreich and Deirdre English have called a "ragtag collection of [other] radical causes" of the time—such as religious revivals, labor organizing, and the improvement of treatment for prisoners and those deemed insane.[13] Women's rights proponents were particularly drawn to the goals of the popular health movement, which included defending women's role as healers, encouraging physical exercise for women, and attacking the restrictiveness of women's clothing, such as the corset. Both popular health movement activists and nineteenth-century feminists appreciated the "traditional role" of women as lay health practitioners, as well as women's capability as informed patients who deserved the ability to choose treatment outside of the medical model.[14] These concerns brought many women together across class and racial lines to support a common general cause.

However, although these diverse constituencies of women were in agreement regarding their dissatisfaction with the heroic measures of nineteenth-century medical physicians—which often included bloodletting and inconsistent dosing of medications, such as calomel (mercury chloride, a potentially lethal mineral compound that was commonly used for fevers), antimony (a toxic natural sulfide used to expel a variety of ailments from the body), and a variety of other emetics, purgatives, and opiates—they were not always in agreement about what or who should be supported in their place.[15] Most working-class white women supported local botanical healers, and most African American women favored herbalists within their communities. Most affluent white women, however, offered their support to the primarily male homeopathic profession that was emerging during the early 1800s.[16] This was widely interpreted as an effort on the part of wealthy white women to distance themselves from the more "radical associations" of the popular health movement—particularly the abolitionists against slavery and the "workingman's movement," composed of small farmers, artisans, and factory workers who were dissatisfied with the capitalist system and the "parasitical" upper class.[17]

Despite these internal tensions, strong coalitions formed among the social reform movements of the time, and there was a good deal of overlap among the people involved in them. With the outbreak of the Civil War in 1861, this meant that activists' attention was focused on the abolitionist movement. Thus, as Baxandall, Gordon, and Reverby have explained, "While economically the Civil War was in some sense a beginning, politically it was in many ways a culmination, even a temporary end, to a period of political activism," bringing about the conclusion of several social movements of the time—including the popular health movement.[18] Although activists associated with this movement did not succeed in keeping biomedicine from dominating healthcare in the twentieth century—and, as some historians argue, the healthcare field was polluted "by quacks and patent medicine peddlers"[19]—it did have some measure of success, along with the women's movement, in its support of the benefits of women's physical exercise and the freedom for women to wear nonrestrictive clothing. Ultimately, the movement's greatest success was that it maintained access to training in various systems of healthcare for working-class people, women, and African Americans into the early 1900s.

In 1910, however, the Flexner Report—the first corporate-funded survey of the quality of North American medical education—generated a strong blow to these victories and resulted in the closure of smaller, poorer, and "irregular" schools throughout the country. In 1906, the Carnegie Foundation initiated the Flexner Report at the American Medical Association's (AMA) recommendation. Businessman Abraham Flexner wrote the report based on his visits to regular, eclectic, homeopathic, and osteopathic schools in the United States and Canada. The report had far-reaching effects, initiating a significant decline in the number of biomedical schools (from 162 in 1906 to only 79 in 1924), requiring surviving irregular schools to orient their curricula toward those of medical schools, and prompting a shift in financial support by corporate-sponsored philanthropies to fund only regular medical schools that were defined in the report as "superior."[20]

Notably, the schools that were most affected by the resulting federal policy changes and selective philanthropic funding were those that admitted women and African Americans, as well as those that offered low-cost training to working-class and lower-middle-class students.[21] As medical anthropologist Hans Baer explains:

> [The Flexner Report] contributed to the drastic change in socioeconomic, ethnic, and gender composition of the regular medical profession. Before the Flexner Report, access to a medical career was relatively open; afterwards it was largely confined to those of the upper and upper-middle classes. In 1910 there were eight medical schools that catered to African Americans as well as a substantial number that primarily served women; the Flexner Report contributed to the closing of all but two of the black medical schools—the one at Howard University in Washington, D.C., and Meharry Medical College in Nashville, Tennessee—and all but one of the women's medical schools.[22]

As biomedicine became more established in the United States during the 1800s, some middle-class white women had also begun to enter the market as "regular" medical physicians. Similar to the women who were involved in the earlier popular health movement, Ehrenreich and English describe the emergence of women in medicine as "motivated by the spirit of reform: they were opposed to the excesses of heroic medicine. . . . The mid-nineteenth century movement of women into medical training took on the aspects of a *crusade*—for female health, for morality, for decency."[23] These women's crusade for healthcare reform *within* the "regular" medical system continued into the twentieth century. Despite the important gains for the middle-class white women who were able to become physicians during this time, their reform efforts also contributed significantly to the increased scrutiny of "morality" and "decency" in women's reproductive practices more broadly, particularly those of African American women and poor women of all colors.[24]

The Fertility Control Debates

A central element in the campaign for feminine morality and decency in the late 1800s was the contentious debate over contraception and abortion. Notably, prior to this time, fertility control techniques were used widely in the United States with little public commentary.[25] During the late 1800s, however, the increasing use of abortion among white married women, the intensifying eugenics movement (which advocated forced sterilizations for women deemed "unfit" to mother by public health officials), the push to further expand the medical profession, and feminists' demands for freedom from male control of their bodies all contributed to the heated debates over governmental regulation of abortion and contraception.

Central to these debates was the dramatic shift in the social profile of women who sought abortions during the nineteenth century. In the early 1800s, women who had abortions (or who were reportedly doing so by the accounts of court cases and physicians' records, since there are no government statistics from this era) were primarily slaves and young white women who had children out of wedlock.[26] Yet by the late 1800s the demand for abortion had shifted largely to women who were married, native-born, educated, Protestant, and from the middle and upper classes.[27] The widespread use of abortion during the late 1800s—estimated by at least one physician to be as high as 20 to 25 percent of pregnancies—was a primary factor in the push to criminalize fertility control.[28] As historian Rickie Solinger has summarized, "Abortion was dangerous because it thinned the population of Anglo-Saxon white people. Abortion risked the racial future of the United States."[29]

Physicians harnessed the growing public outrage over high rates of abortion to fuel campaigns that would further restrict the practice of irregular practitioners, many of whom were the primary providers of abortions at that time.[30] Physicians who criticized midwives (particularly immigrant midwives in the North) also charged that these women were guilty of providing abortions.[31] Although this was true in some cases, physicians highlighted the "criminality" of midwives and downplayed the abortions provided by other physicians during the time in an effort to discredit midwives and encourage women to abandon their care in favor of the growing profession of obstetrics. Further, as women's health researcher Carol Weisman notes, "The declining birth rate is likely to have posed a serious threat to the livelihood of physicians, who depended on attending deliveries, and to have contributed to their attempts to control the market for women's health care."[32] Political scientist Rosalind

Petchesky has also explained that lobbying *against* abortion contributed to the physicians' "push to monopolize the market in health and childbirth, a particularly female market."[33] In 1859, the AMA passed a resolution condemning abortion, urging legislators to become involved in the prohibition of both abortion and contraception.[34] By associating immorality and "unnaturalness" with both irregular practitioners and women who sought abortions, physicians were successful in creating a cultural milieu in which abortion came to signify what anthropologist Faye Ginsburg has described as "a disruption of harmonious domestic relations and the social order in general."[35] Interestingly, physicians' emphasis on morality and domesticity in their crusade against abortion made for an "unlikely circumstantial alliance" with nineteenth-century feminists.[36]

By the late 1800s, feminists had begun to organize around a variety of issues, including women's suffrage, better access to education, improved access to medical services, and the elimination of abortion. In contrast to the association of feminists with pro-choice struggles during the late 1900s, many native-born, white, affluent women in the nineteenth century became strong supporters of the womanly duty to bear children. Indeed, well-known nineteenth-century proponent of women's rights, Elizabeth Cady Stanton, called abortion "the degradation of women," though she argued that "voluntary motherhood"—through access to birth control and the legal ability to say no to her husband's sexual demands—was the key to women's salvation.[37] However, nineteenth-century feminists disagreed with physicians' accusations that *only* women were selfish and "abnormal" for shirking their motherly responsibilities.[38] Instead, feminists feared that the availability of birth control and abortion services would encourage male promiscuity, contribute to the loss of women's control over their bodies and morality to men, and diminish husbands' commitment to their families.[39]

In contrast, other feminists became proponents of birth control during the early 1900s. Most famously, Margaret Sanger, who founded the American Birth Control League (which later became known as Planned Parenthood), advocated women's control over their fertility as a means of social mobility and persuaded many middle-class women, both white and African American, to support access to birth control.[40] Ironically, however, as historian Jean Matthews has documented, "Most of the thousands of letters that Sanger received came from working-class women, telling their stories and begging for help, but most of the people who joined various birth-control leagues were middle-class, often professional men and women."[41] Despite the interracial interest Sanger was able to generate for birth control among middle-class women, she and other white organizers ultimately alienated many African American supporters when they built alliances with the population control establishment, which promoted eugenic goals of selective breeding under the framework of public health.[42] As

Solinger has argued, "Planned Parenthood and other organizations contributed to early efforts to define motherhood as a class privilege. Purposefully or not, these groups gave force to the idea that poor women, especially women of color, should be targets of centrally planned reproductive control, not bearers of reproductive rights."[43]

At the turn of the twentieth century, the eugenic movement was becoming increasingly concerned with the 50 percent decline in the birthrate among white women from 1800 to 1900—from 7.04 to 3.56.[44] Influenced by the eugenic sentiments developing in Germany at the time, U.S. nationalists suggested that strategic population control efforts could contribute to the propagation of "the white race."[45] Population control officials suggested that by promoting contraception (and sterilization) among immigrants, women of color, and poor women, and encouraging pregnancies among white middle-class and affluent women, a "better," more "pure" race would be the result.[46] Consequently, eugenics proponents became a primary source of funding for fertility control clinics in the United States, which led to controversial alliances between feminists struggling to ensure access to birth control for a broad range of women and eugenicists who hoped that these technologies would limit births among poor and nonwhite women. As Gordon explains in *Woman's Body, Woman's Right*:

> Most birth-control clinics appreciated the eugenists' support for disseminating contraceptives in the absence of pathological indications. The clinics also acceded to eugenists' research interests. Many clinics conducted inquiries into the hereditary histories of their patients and presumably advised the women as to the desirability of having children[47]. . . . A review of the work of seventy birth-control clinics in Britain and the United States, published in 1930, proudly demonstrated that they had reached a disproportionately large number of working-class women, and claimed a eugenic effect from doing so.[48]

As a result, middle-class African American women began to organize instead through their own community networks,[49] both for access to fertility control and against the compulsory sterilization of many African American women. Loretta Ross, reproductive rights activist and former program director for the National Black Women's Health Project, has noted that "a clear sense of dual or 'paired' values also emerged among African-American women: to want individual control over their bodies while simultaneously resisting government and private depopulation policies that blurred the distinction between incentives and coercion.[50] African-American women supported birth control, but at the same time they offered a strong critique of eugenicists."[51] This support of fertility control was not unanimous, however, and many African American women continued to resist birth control into the 1900s, arguing that it was an attempt at genocide, designed to reduce the size of the black population.[52] In a peculiarly related development, physicians associated with the national eugenics movement also joined feminists as proponents of the use of pain medication in childbirth as a way of encouraging affluent white women (who could afford access to the emerging technology) to give birth in larger numbers and in the hospital.

The Movement for Twilight Sleep

A benchmark of emancipation for many affluent white women during the early 1900s was access to pain medication in childbirth.[53] The campaign for access to twilight sleep in labor—an injection of morphine and the amnesiac drug scopolamine, which would ensure a "painless childbirth"—drew increased attention to the promises of hospital birth. At the turn of the twentieth century, German doctors developed twilight sleep, which allowed a woman to remain semi-conscious during labor—at least inasmuch as she could respond to instructions—but to have little or no memory of her childbirth experience. Additionally, to achieve success with twilight sleep, the patient had to be monitored frequently by nurses or physicians and placed in an environment that provided little external visual or auditory stimulation.[54]

Initially, American physicians rejected the treatment as unsafe, unreliable, and too demanding of their time, but affluent women who could afford access to this new amenity were so excited about the prospect of a pain-free childbirth that a popular campaign was initiated to gain access to the procedure.[55] As women's health researcher Margarete Sandelowski has explained, "The Twilight Sleep debate of 1914–1915 was not simply an argument about the advantages and disadvantages of a pain-relieving regimen but rather a lay revolt against what was perceived as the medical expropriation of knowledge belonging to the people."[56] This lay campaign solidified feminist and suffragist aims to unite many white women—who had access to hospitals and could frequently afford twilight sleep—around a common cause, demanding freedom from the suffering of childbirth as a way to emancipate women.[57] In contrast to the ways arguments over fertility control had divided feminist organizing efforts because of religious and political differences, historian Judith Walzer Leavitt has noted that the "upper- and middle-class clubwomen" who led the struggle for twilight sleep argued that the movement drew women together around "childbirth as an experience that united all women."[58]

However, this movement also drew attention to the class and race inequities that had begun to further segregate access to these new childbirth services by the early 1900s. Prior to the turn of the twentieth century and the advent of commercial markets for childbirth, women's reproductive options in the United States were largely the same.[59] Women of all races and classes gave birth at home—most often with midwives—before the widespread use of hospitals for "confinement" during pregnancy.[60] In the South, both white and black women relied on African American midwives. In the North, women sought midwives who were recent immigrants from European countries with various degrees of midwifery training outside of North America. It was only during the intensified growth of the medical profession during the late 1800s and early 1900s that more diverse childbirth options became available for some women.

As these new options were becoming available, one physician wrote in 1929: "To allow a mother to go through the so-called natural birth experience without such relief as we may give from suffering is the most inhuman and unkind thing."[61] Not surprisingly, however, scholars of color, such as Gertrude Fraser, have aptly noted that "doctors were willing to dim their sense of outrage [for poor and African American women] about the supposed cruelty of natural childbirth."[62] Notably, working-class white women were also initially attracted to twilight sleep and saw it as a way to decrease maternal and infant mortality and increase "vitality among the mothers of children,"[63] though many were also fearful that it would remain a "superadded luxury of the wealthy mother."[64] Indeed, physicians routinely denied pain medication to poorer women who were unable to afford it and who were considered less needy of pain relief because of their supposed higher tolerance for pain.[65]

Ultimately, physicians embraced twilight sleep to enhance the profession of obstetrics and to encourage affluent white women to give birth in the hospital. Historians Richard Wertz and Dorothy Wertz have noted that both eugenicists and doctors "could not fail to notice that, if such women ['wealthy society ladies' and 'well-dressed mothers'] once more regarded delivery as a joyful experience, the Anglo-Saxon race would not 'die out,' and women might rediscover the joys of traditional femininity and maternity."[66] A 1915 editorial in a popular women's journal touted the advantages of twilight sleep: "The twentieth century woman will no more think of having an ordinary practitioner attend her in childbed at home. She will go to a hospital as a matter of course."[67]

Reform Efforts to Improve Maternal and Infant Healthcare

With the increasing public scrutiny of childbirth practices at the turn of the twentieth century, the improvement of maternal and child healthcare became a primary political concern for various constituencies of women. Working-class

white women and "farm mothers" were becoming increasingly concerned about
the large numbers of deaths among women and children in their communities.[68] Likewise, African American women of all classes sought to improve the
health conditions in their communities and "wanted to offer their children increased access to the medical care that had been so long denied their race."[69]
Middle-class and affluent white feminists, particularly in the northern states,
also became concerned with child safety and emphasized the responsibility of
women from all socioeconomic backgrounds to improve the health of their
children "with expert guidance in the tasks of motherhood" from women's
groups and ultimately a federal agency dedicated to the improvement of maternal and child health.[70] Many women in this later group used their influence
with popular magazines, such as *Good Housekeeping* and *Harper's Monthly
Magazine,* as a strategic political tactic to make their voices heard on a national
level. Many were also suffragists and hoped to bring about healthcare change
through governmental reform.[71] In fact, historian Richard Shryock has noted
that "the crusade for women's health was related both in cause and effect to
the demand for women's rights in general, and the health and feminist movements become indistinguishable at this point."[72]

Through their struggle for suffrage, middle-class and affluent white women
were becoming a persuasive political force on a national level. The lobbying efforts of what sociologist and political scientist Theda Skocpol has described as
the "women reformers and widespread associations of married women," resulted in Congress passing the Sheppard-Towner Maternal and Infancy Protection Act in 1921, which became "America's first explicit federal social welfare
legislation."[73] The federal matching grants managed by the Children's Bureau
funded a variety of services, including: (1) the deployment of public health nurses
to offer prenatal care and childbirth education in expectant mothers' homes; (2)
the improvement of accurate birth statistics; (3) the establishment of prenatal
clinics and infant welfare centers staffed by physicians and nurses; (4) the in-
spection of hospitals and laboratories; (5) the promotion of birth registration;
and (6) the licensure, supervision, and instruction of midwives.

The passage of the Nineteenth Amendment, which gave women the right
to vote in 1920, and the introduction of the Sheppard-Towner Act in 1921 gave
female proponents of maternal and infant healthcare improvements a distinct
political advantage, even over the growing power of the AMA, which strongly
opposed the Sheppard-Towner Act, viewing it as a harbinger of socialized medicine and governmental control of medical services.[74] As historian William Chafe
has explained, "No other event demonstrated so dramatically the eagerness of
politicians to win over the unknown quantity introduced into the electorate by
the enactment of the Nineteenth Amendment."[75] Attesting to the growing
political power of these women's groups, all states, with the exception of

Massachusetts, where the AMA's lobby was the strongest, accepted Sheppard-Towner Act grants.[76] In fact, Wertz and Wertz note in *Lying-In* that a New York governor who initially rejected the federal grant, but spent a similar sum on a new hog barn for the state fairgrounds, was defeated during the next election following a strong campaign by women's organizations that "publicized his preference for the health of swine over that of children."[77]

One side effect of affluent women's organizing to encourage the passage of the Sheppard-Towner Act was that social reformers opened up the homes of the poor to increased government scrutiny and ultimately initiated legislative intervention into childbirth and childcare.[78] In fact, government interests were a key factor in the new state and federal concerns with the welfare of mothers and children. Sally Austen Tom, nurse-midwife and women's health historian, has explained, "Even though World War I was justified as 'the war to end all wars,' the government was insuring itself for future wars by ploughing money into public health. For the first time children were recognized as future members of the military and thus deserving of federal funds. Similarly, women were recognized as producers of future fighting men, and their health became a national resource."[79] Indeed, 33 percent of all men examined for military service during World War I (1914–1918) were disqualified because of physical defects,[80] which prompted grave concerns over the development of "well-born" and "useful" citizens.[81] New methods of assessment were also coming into vogue in the early 1900s, such as the IQ test, which "became a tool for determining which child could become a good citizen, a good soldier, a good worker, a legitimate reproducer, and which child should not have been born to begin with."[82] Of course, these distinctions frequently mimicked familiar racialized and class-based hierarchies.

Thus it is not surprising that the improvement of maternal and infant healthcare was hardly a uniform experience for all women. For instance, many healthcare reformers considered the decline of homebirth in the United States a marker of healthcare improvement in the early twentieth century. However, although "progress" toward hospital births appeared steady in national statistics—only 5 percent of births occurred in the hospital in 1900,[83] but by 1938 the number was close to 50 percent, up to 95 percent in 1955,[84] and 99 percent from 1980 to the present[85]—nonwhite women were far more likely to still be giving birth at home than their white counterparts. In 1936, for example, North Carolina reported that 67.4 percent of all nonwhite deliveries were attended by midwives in the home, as opposed to 11.4 percent of all white deliveries.[86] A variety of factors contributed to this racial split, most importantly the restrictions on hospital care for women of color that remained in place in many areas until the Civil Rights Act in 1964. Although in the early 1900s hospital stays for childbirth were touted as "vacations" for well-to-do women,[87] literary scholar Valerie Lee has observed in *Granny Midwives and Black Women Writers* that "they were not recreational for black women who, due to Jim Crow laws, were admitted to basement wards or segregated wings. Nor were they initially desirable for poor women who lost what little autonomy and control they had."[88] Attesting to this racial and socioeconomic divide, African American women and poor women were disproportionately subjected to the over 70,000 eugenic sterilizations of "unfit" mothers in the United States, which occurred in hospitals during the early to mid-1900s.[89]

Thus much like the contradictions African Americans faced regarding their support of or opposition to fertility control in the early 1900s,[90] a sense of dual values was emerging among women of color and recent immigrants to the United States, those who sought equal access to quality medical care but at the same time valued the services of the local midwives in their communities. For African American and Mexican American communities in the South and for the recent immigrants from southern and eastern Europe in the North, midwives were often the only healthcare providers that poor women could afford.[91] Wertz and Wertz have further explained:

> Midwives were obviously attractive to many people, for they usually charged much less than a doctor and often provided such other services as housecleaning, laundry, and postnatal care of the mother and child for several days, while the more expensive doctor usually attended only the birth. . . . Many [immigrant women] disliked clinics, which marked them as charity cases, and most could afford a midwife. Hospital birth was not part of their tradition, nor was the attendance of a man during birth.[92]

Many poor women and women of color also sought midwives because they were less likely to harbor prejudices about the class, race, and ethnic backgrounds of their clients. American studies scholar Molly Ladd-Taylor has written: "Expectant mothers could count on midwives when doctors refused to treat them because of prejudice, bad roads, or inability to pay."[93] Further, African American midwives, who were often referred to as "granny midwives," were central figures in their communities.[94] As one recent childbirth education guide, which was written for African American women, recounts, "Grannies, as they were affectionately called, were much more than women who came to 'catch' babies. They were dieticians, psychologists, loan officers, sex therapists, prayer partners, marriage counselors, and friends to the women they attended."[95]

Despite the racialized and class-based healthcare inequities that the Sheppard-Towner Act reinforced, some authors have touted the act as the most successful achievement of midwifery proponents in the early 1900s.[96] More specifically, it was successful for affluent and middle-class white women who desired access to the hospital and to "upgrade" midwifery services, often in the form of nurse-midwives, but for the poor immigrant and African American midwives practicing during that time the act had more negative effects. For instance, it undermined local respect for elderly midwives in African American communities by favoring younger midwives who were perceived by government and medical officials as being more compliant with federal and local mandates. It also instituted a fee-for-service standard that disrupted reciprocal community networks and established formerly independent midwifery practices under the supervision of health departments.[97] Fraser has described the legislation starkly, as "an ambitious venture to colonize and civilize African American midwives and mothers."[98]

Ultimately, the Sheppard-Towner Act joined with several other cultural shifts to contribute to the elimination of lay midwives in the United States during the twentieth century. Anthropologist Holly Mathews has explained in "Killing the Medical Self-Help Tradition among African Americans":

> Several independent events in the 1920s would act together to lead to the rapid decline of the lay midwife. These included the application of increasingly stringent regulations to midwives by local health boards, the passage by Congress of restrictive immigration acts that limited the number of new midwives arriving in the country, and changing attitudes on the part of the upper-middle classes favoring smaller family size and increasing medical intervention in birth as a sign of progressive social attitudes. . . . [This] division of interests . . . split women along the lines of class and race.[99]

As a result of fervent physician opposition to midwives and the incorporation of ideas about hygiene that necessitated childbirth in the hospital, much of the healthcare reform legislation that was initially intended to train midwives became the means through which they were denied licenses or chose to stop practicing because of increased government surveillance.

For example, Ladd-Taylor has described the experience of African American midwives in the South during instructional trainings for midwives, funded by grants from the Children's Bureau following the Sheppard-Towner Act:

> The Children's Bureau tried to provide adequate services for all racial and ethnic groups throughout the country. Convinced that education and research would lead to action, the Bureau staff expected the instructional programs of the Sheppard-Towner Act to convince

midwives and mothers to reject the "superstitious" practices of the past in favor of new procedures approved by the medical establishment. Well-intentioned but culturally insensitive, most Sheppard-Towner nurses had little respect for rural black culture or traditional healing. Although they believed they were helping rural mothers and protecting midwives, their attempts to make midwifery scientific and professional denied the value of traditional skills and folk healing, thus furthering the medicalization of birth.[100]

During this time, some African American midwives engaged in resistant acts, or what Fraser has called "microbehaviors," to sabotage the medical management of their bodies, such as continuing to employ techniques taught by elders during labor and birth when medical officials were not present.[101] Often, however, the same women who resisted medicalization through the use of traditional childbirth techniques also found ways to incorporate health practices that they found useful and advantageous to improving maternal and infant mortality rates.[102] Overall, however, the medical and legislative efforts to eliminate midwives in the early 1900s met with little organized resistance. Midwife Margaret Charles Smith's and women's health researcher Linda Janet Holmes's research on midwifery in Alabama suggests that the existing midwifery clubs of the time worked primarily with local health departments to offer refresher courses and social events, and that civil rights organizations did not rally around midwives.[103] Fraser has further argued that the promise of a share in the "medical progress" around childbirth in the early 1900s "helped to subvert organized protest among disenfranchised and impoverished African Americans," as well as other marginalized groups.[104]

While efforts toward medicalization had set the wheels in motion to eliminate African American midwives, white women's political organizing declined in the late 1920s and women did not remain a coherent political lobby, in part because they did not all agree upon how to best improve maternal and infant healthcare.[105] Coupled with the fact that the AMA had become an even more powerful lobby against governmental control of medicine, the Sheppard-Towner Act was terminated in 1929. Legislators became less concerned about a cohesive "women's voting bloc" throughout the 1920s, particularly as it became evident that women had a variety of interests and concerns that influenced their votes.[106] Thus, in *Reclaiming Birth*, Margot Edwards and Mary Waldorf have explained that congressmen were content to shift federal and state healthcare priorities away from maternal and infant healthcare "when doctors convinced legislators that childbirth was a disease, and, therefore, properly their province."[107]

As a result, a good deal of women's organizing around reproductive health issues during the remainder of the twentieth century focused on local struggles for healthcare access, challenged state healthcare policies, and demanded access to reproductive services on a community level.[108] Although the debate over the legalization of abortion both before and after the *Roe v. Wade* decision in 1973 mobilized women to become politically involved at a national level, women's efforts to gain (and to restrict) access to abortion services existed mainly within their own communities.[109] Another example of a nationally recognized movement where major gains for women's reproductive rights were primarily made locally is the natural childbirth movement, which I discuss at length in the following chapter. For instance, although literature on "natural childbirth" methods and critiques of medicalized childbirth made the goals of the movement available on a national (and an international) scale, policy changes in state laws and in particular hospitals were almost always the result of community-based grassroots organizing.

2

The Birth of Consumer Activism for Midwives

From the Natural Childbirth Movement to
Recent Legislative Efforts

The home-birth movement across the United States
represents an extraordinary and sometimes uneasy alliance
of feminist and traditionalist women and men. For the
feminists, childbirth tends to be one of many fronts on
which the struggle for women's control of their lives is
taking place. For the traditionalists, the childbirth issue is
rooted in the context of the traditional wife-mother role.
—BARBARA KATZ ROTHMAN, *IN LABOR*, 2ND EDITION

As the natural childbirth movement gained popular support during the
1950s, it drew together a religiously and politically diverse array of
women who had become dissatisfied with medically managed childbirth after labor and delivery care moved from the home to the hospital in
the early 1900s. Despite the decline of the natural childbirth movement in the
1980s, many of the goals and resistant strategies of its proponents have en-
dured, and midwifery and homebirth are now available in many U.S. communities. As explained in the Introduction, no "official" name has emerged for this
contemporary movement, largely because struggles for access to midwives
became increasingly localized, following the broader trend toward community-
based efforts in the natural childbirth movement. Recently, however, national
organizations for midwives and groups such as the Big Push for Midwives and
the MAMA Campaign are attempting to unite local movements in an effort
to promote the right to access midwives throughout the United States.

This chapter provides an overview of this history but also an alternative to
uniform portrayals of the "history of midwifery" that have placed U.S. midwives and their supporters in a seamless account of "sisters in struggle." I join
other feminist historians and social scientists in their efforts to acknowledge

that no "single history" of midwifery exists but, rather, that overlapping, and sometimes distinct, histories have been punctuated by the race and class inequities described in Chapter 1.[1] As historian Lesley Biggs has reflected regarding the initial history of midwifery and childbirth in Ontario that she wrote in the 1980s (which focused on "allopathic medicine's attempts to gain a monopoly over health care and that female midwives were a source of unwanted competition"), it is not so much what feminist historians *have* said but what they *have not* said in terms of women's diverse experiences of childbirth.[2] I agree that the detrimental impact of patriarchal medicine on midwifery is important, and it has been well documented. In this chapter I broaden this discussion to better address how women's (and midwives') differing experiences with reproduction and state regulation continued to produce different goals for improving childbirth into the twenty-first century. This is particularly relevant to the emergence of a self-conscious "consumer"-driven movement for midwives,[3] which draws renewed attention to the continued socioeconomic disparities among homebirth mothers. As we saw in the previous chapter, Americans' cultural understandings of motherhood and their expectations about reproductive healthcare have not remained static or universal, and this has been equally true since the beginning of the natural childbirth movement. As Rickie Solinger's broader historical research on reproductive politics demonstrates:

> Definitions [of motherhood] have . . . changed over time and have been applied to different groups of women differently, depending on their race and class. . . . [Yet] social and legal rules have historically governed who can be a legitimate mother, under what circumstances, and how women can and cannot manage their fertility. These rules have always been linked to traditional assumptions about women's "natural work" as mothers.[4]

Accordingly, this chapter also examines how debates over the shifting definitions of "natural," "primitive," and "normal" birth often illustrate (and reproduce) profoundly different experiences and expectations for childbearing women. I conclude with an overview of how contemporary organizing for midwives and homebirth remains punctuated by these differences.

The Natural Childbirth Movement

As a result of the steady decline in childbirth-related mortality in the United States during the 1920s and 1930s, public attention to childbirth shifted from mothers' mere survival to concerns regarding women's satisfaction and comfort during the labor and delivery process.[5] During the 1940s and 1950s, many middle-class and affluent white women were becoming disillusioned with the promises of "painless" childbirth under anesthesia and what had been touted as "vacations" to modern hospitals for childbirth.[6] These women began to read about childbirth methods that were being developed in Europe in books such as Grantley Dick-Read's *Childbirth without Fear* in 1944 and *No Time for Fear* in 1955, from Britain, and Ferdinand Lamaze's *Painless Childbirth* in 1956, from France, which encouraged women to give birth without anesthesia.[7] These authors considered childbirth a "naturally" painless event and suggested Pavlovian techniques to condition reflexes to raise a woman's pain threshold; thus, as anthropologist Sheila Kitzinger summarized in *The Experience of Childbirth*, "Sensations formerly interpreted by the brain as painful are accepted as painless."[8] These techniques were initially known in the United States as "psychoprophylaxis" and "prepared childbirth"[9] but they became more widely recognized among expectant American mothers as the Lamaze method of "rigorous breathing" through contractions, particularly after the 1959 publication *Thank You, Dr. Lamaze*, describing American mother Marjorie Karmel's personal childbirth journey to Paris to have her baby with Dr. Lamaze.[10]

As these techniques gained popularity in the 1960s and 1970s, women began to form local consciousness-raising groups to explore natural childbirth methods, departing from the original literature that had been written almost entirely by men, which included, as sociologist Robbie Pfeufer Kahn has critiqued, "little palpable sense of the women themselves [or] of human agency."[11] One of the better-known (and still popular) groups was the La Leche League (LLL), founded in 1956. Members of LLL urged women to breastfeed their babies, challenging doctors' orders to feed babies formula and questioning the interests of the growing formula industry. As Pamela Klassen has explained, "Reworking an older maternalist movement that had supported 'scientific motherhood,' La Leche League emphasized that the mother—not her doctor—knew her baby and her own body best."[12]

Two other enduring national organizations for natural childbirth began in 1960. Marjorie Karmel, Elizabeth Bing, and Elly Rakowitz founded the American Society for Psychoprophylaxis in Obstetrics (ASPO), based on the Lamaze method. In a recent interview, Bing described their work retrospectively as "a consumer movement . . . a time when the public doubted everything their parents had done."[13] Yet however consumer-driven it was, ASPO also remained in close company with the medical profession in an effort to disarm the "opponent . . . by an offer of partnership."[14] Alternatively, the International Childbirth Education Association (ICEA), a national federation of local natural childbirth support groups, was more "consumer-based" than ASPO and relied on feminist ideals of "choice" in its motto "Freedom of Choice Based on Knowledge of Alternatives."[15] Kahn explains in *Bearing Meaning* that ICEA's "parent activists chose professional consultants whose viewpoints tended to lie outside mainstream medicine, such as Margaret Mead and Ashley Montagu."[16] Anthropologists, such as Mead and Montagu, played a central role in the natural childbirth movement during the 1960s and 1970s, prompting proponents to examine the birth practices of women in non-Western cultures.[17] Although the anthropological record of cross-cultural variation in childbirth since the late 1800s has been roundly critiqued for its racist and colonial assumptions,[18] it nevertheless made a strong argument that there were indeed alternatives to the "advancement" of childbirth through medical intervention.[19]

For instance, Sheila Kitzinger's *Women as Mothers*, published in 1978, demonstrated to both popular and scholarly audiences that Western birthing practices were indeed as subjective and culturally bound as those in other cultures.[20] Anthropologist Brigitte Jordan, widely touted as the midwife to the anthropology of reproduction, also produced in 1978 the first comparative ethnography of childbirth, *Birth in Four Cultures*.[21] Jordan carefully highlighted the distinction between parturition (the act of childbearing) and childbirth itself, "the culture-specific social matrix within which human biology is embedded."[22] Addressing the return to a more "traditional" form of childbirth espoused by many natural childbirth advocates, Jordan offered a model of "mutual accommodation" to value both indigenous birth practices and the exportation of practical Western technological developments. Natural childbirth proponents drew on these and other anthropological studies of childbirth to challenge the uniformity and supposed superiority of the "civilized" reproductive practices suggested by the medical model.

As the natural childbirth movement reached its height in the 1960s and 1970s, childbirth reform efforts to change policies in many hospitals were in full swing. Activists petitioned hospitals and physicians to allow family to be with the pregnant woman during labor and delivery, demanded childbirth with less medication and interventions,[23] and encouraged mother and newborn bonding and breastfeeding. Ultimately, childbearing women began to shift the public and medical emphasis on eliminating women's pain during labor and delivery to a focus on "pleasure" in the childbirth process. As Margarete Sandelowski has explained: "Professional literature indicated that it was the 'consumer' who was 'rebelling' against the way in which obstetrics was being practiced and demanding more personalized treatment."[24] This "consumer rebellion" for childbirth reform within the hospital (among women who could afford to make choices about where and with whom they would give birth) was a largely a success; many hospitals began to allow fathers and other family members into delivery rooms, physicians and nurses intervened less (for example, by reducing the routine use of enemas and forceps), and labor and delivery units began to provide a more "homelike" environment for birthcare.

Yet some natural childbirth proponents were still not satisfied with what they considered perfunctory and superficial changes to the medical model of childbirth in U.S. hospitals.[25] Indeed, as sociologist Barbara Katz Rothman has argued, when natural childbirth preparation styles, such as those advocated by Dick-Read and Lamaze, were introduced to American women, they were primarily used in an effort to reform existing hospital birthing practices, not to radically challenge American assumptions about birth.[26] In the 1960s and 1970s, a subset of the natural childbirth movement began to reconsider homebirth as an alternative to medically managed childbirth. As sociologists Deborah Sullivan and Rose Weitz explain in *Labor Pains*:

> By the late 1960s, an increasing number of women were strongly committed to and had prepared for a family-centered natural childbirth. They often suffered disappointment, however, when hospital staff, a substitute physician, or even their own personal physician overrode their choice and refused fathers entry to the delivery, ordered heavier sedation and labor augmentation, or cut an episiotomy. Recognizing the limits on true reform within hospitals, the most disenchanted started choosing home birth. These individuals believe[d] that they [would] never gain sufficient control within hospitals to replace the active medical management of a passive "diseased" patient with a more holistic, wellness model that stresse[d] self-responsibility, family involvement, and minimal medical intervention.[27]

To support the emergent homebirth movement, organizations promoting alternatives to the medical model of childbirth proliferated during the 1970s. In fact, one study showed that between 1973 and 1976, at least a dozen national and regional organizations were founded to support homebirth.[28] Groups such as the National Association of Parents and Professionals for Safe Alternatives in Childbirth (NAPSAC),[29] the American College of Home Obstetrics (ACHO), Informed Homebirth, and the Association for Childbirth at Home International (ACHI) formed a solid base for education and cooperation among homebirth proponents. These groups were also instrumental in popularizing other alternatives to the medical management of childbirth in the hospital during the 1970s, such as birth centers operated by midwives.

By the late 1970s, the broader natural childbirth movement had begun to wane, largely because of many women's "consumer satisfaction" with hospital-based improvements in maternity care. Notably, however, these successes were not universal, particularly for working-class and poor women, who continued to experience higher levels of medical intervention than their middle-class and affluent counterparts. Low-income women were not able to "consume" costly services and products, such as childbirth classes and self-help guides for childbirth preparation, and clinic clients were not offered a choice of doctors or the luxury of rejecting technological interventions.[30] Ultimately, the ability to control the circumstances of childbirth remained largely with middle-class white women.[31] Within the movement for homebirth, the success of activists from different classes and racial backgrounds was also uneven. Judith Walzer Leavitt has described how "class and ethnicity factors" worked against the childbirth reform efforts of low-income women and one multiracial coalition of activists:

> When the poor women of Chicago's inner city, many of whom were Hispanic and Black, tried to organize to save the home birth service of the Chicago Maternity Center, they were not successful in presenting their case about the importance of birth options. The closing of the Center in 1974, despite public protests from the women who had utilized or who wanted to utilize the service that Joseph DeLee had started in 1895, indicates that women, even when acting in unison, cannot always win their way.[32]

Despite growing interest in homebirth and midwifery during the 1970s and 1980s, the natural childbirth movement was winding down by the 1980s and 1990s, and this had a detrimental effect on midwives who promoted natural childbirth outside of the hospital. As sociologist Raymond De Vries explains in *Making Midwives Legal*:

> The failure of the alternative birth movement fell hardest on midwives. It was their hope to establish themselves as independent professionals, emulating the model of midwifery care found in some European nations. Instead, they were forced either to become a part of the world of obstetrics or to be content with a peripheral role, living in the shadow of questionable legitimacy. Nurse-midwives chose the former strategy, working under the supervision of physicians. This decision gave them a legitimate place in American medicine, but it led to accusations of selling out and co-optation. "Lay" midwives did not sell out. They refused formal education based in obstetric science and avoided entanglement in medical hierarchies. They retained their purity but were dismissed as countercultural throwbacks in a world moving away from the libertarian excesses of the sixties toward the

staid conformism of the Reagan-Bush eighties. Midwifery, with the promise of a more natural view of birth, seemed destined to remain nothing more than an anomaly in America.[33]

Yet the push for midwives and homebirth had not ended in the United States. Rather, like many long-term social and political movements, the struggle for natural childbirth became what social movement theorists have called a "movement in abeyance," one that temporarily suspended large-scale action but nevertheless remobilized into the upsurge of activism for "alternative birth," midwives, and homebirth during the 1990s and into the twenty-first century.[34] The struggles within the movement, particularly over political and religious diversity, have maintained a significant influence on the strategies that organizers have adopted, even in recent years.

Uniting Strange Bedfellows: Political and Religious Diversity

As the natural childbirth movement shifted from its initial Christian focus on the religious importance of natural childbirth to associations with the countercultural, consumer, and feminist movements of the 1960s, the diversity of interest in natural childbirth became both a strategic advantage and a potentially divisive characteristic of the movement. Beginning in the 1940s, Christian childbirth activists were central to childbirth reform efforts in the United States.[35] The natural childbirth manuals that gained popularity in the 1940s and 1950s, such as those by British obstetrician Grantley Dick-Read,[36] proclaimed that natural childbirth was a way for a woman to confirm what Klassen has described in *Blessed Events* as "her God-given role as a mother."[37] In one of the earliest how-to texts for homebirth, Patricia Cloyd Carter peppered her political critique of medicalized childbirth—as well as her call for socialized medicine and the invocation of Lucina, the "Goddess of Childbirth"—with biblical allusions and references to God.[38] Into the 1960s, Christian childbirth activists such as Helen Wessel revived Dick-Read's biblical focus on childbirth and argued that the family pastor was as important to preparation for childbirth as the physician.[39]

As the natural childbirth movement gained wider recognition in the 1960s, proponents became associated with the "countercultural" movement. A particularly influential figure during this time was Ina May Gaskin, a midwife who began delivering babies in the back of a VW bus when she joined the "Caravan" in 1970, a "hippie" group that toured the country promoting intentional living.[40] The Caravan eventually settled in Tennessee and formed the commune known as "the Farm." Gaskin established the Farm Midwifery Center there, where women still travel from around the world to give birth and midwives continue to come for training in out-of-hospital birth techniques.[41] Gaskin published *Spiritual Midwifery* in 1975, which emphasized the spiritual aspects of the birth process.[42] This book remains one of the most widely read birth manuals among both midwives and mothers.[43] Gaskin has remained a strong public advocate of midwives, and she continues to embody the "countercultural" roots that precipitated the stereotype of the "hippie" homebirther during the 1960s and 1970s.[44] As sociologist and women's health researcher Margaret Reid has described:

> The countercultural movement was primarily composed of middle-class women and men who had rejected mainstream American institutions in favor of a return to a more natural style of living that embraced values and beliefs that were the antithesis of those of an achievement-oriented culture. Their approach to food and clothing, as well as their belief in a more spiritual approach to life, were reflected in their life style, which appeared to have emerged from a combination of political radicalism and an attraction to Eastern religious zeal. Couples wishing to live by their principles had home births.[45]

Yet demographic research on homebirth during this time indicated a broader makeup of natural childbirth proponents. For example, Lester Hazell, in her study of homebirthers in the San Francisco Bay area during the 1960s and 1970s, found that only about 10 percent of the 300 couples she studied could be identified as "hippies."[46] She described the majority of homebirthers as "typically middle class," women who lived in single-family homes, owned at least one car, were employed, were not on welfare, were not members of an ethnic minority group, and had no household servants.[47] In addition, Hazell emphasized the attitudinal similarities of homebirth proponents: "One of the characteristics of this group is a hard-to-define level of self-awareness which manifests itself in an individual concern for proper nutrition and a kitchen stocked with health food, personal libraries dealing with religious topics, philosophy, positive health, and humanistic psychology."[48]

The natural childbirth movement as a whole was also characterized as part of the broader "consumer movement" or "consumer revolt" of what women's health researcher Sheryl Ruzek has described as "women, students, minorities, service workers, and some segments of the educated elite who [were] concerned with 'public interest' issues (for example, Nader's 'raiders')."[49] As such, middle-class women—who had started to refer to themselves as consumers, to differentiate themselves from childbirth professionals, such as midwives or physicians—were increasingly demanding control over their childbirth and healthcare experiences. Women's word-of-mouth networks and support from many popular print media sources became hallmarks of the natural childbirth "craze."[50]

Some natural childbirth proponents also emphasized associations with feminist organizing efforts during the 1960s. For example, linguist Paula Treichler has pointed out, "Feminists have generally emphasized the woman's right to be informed, fully conscious, and to experience childbirth as a 'natural' process."[51] And journalist Tina Cassidy has written, "It took . . . the force of the women's movement to push back on the outdated stereotypes, to call for reform, and to help some women understand why midwives are better than doctors for attending low-risk births."[52] It is worth remembering, however, as discussed in Chapter 1, that feminists were the ones who initially lobbied *for* medication in childbirth to "free" women from the burden of pain in the early 1900s.

Indeed, feminist support of homebirth and midwives has been spotty, even in recent decades. It was only in 1999 that the National Organization for Women (NOW) issued a resolution to expand "reproductive freedom" to include the support of women's choice to homebirth and to seek midwives as their birthcare providers.[53] This delayed concern over women's rights *during* childbirth is in part why many homebirthers have distanced themselves from the feminist movement for reproductive rights. Many natural childbirth proponents felt belittled by feminists and reproductive rights activists over their concerns about women's rights as mothers. As journalist Jennifer Block has written:

> Mainstream feminist groups have been slow to recognize the right *to* reproduce along with the right to be free *from* reproducing. A focus of the second-wave women's movement was shaking off motherhood as what solely defined womanhood. So perhaps there has been a reluctance to watch over the process that makes women mothers.[54]

Natural childbirth advocates' and homebirthers' frustration with the lack of feminist response in defense of women's choices *during* childbirth paralleled the discontent among many women of color in the 1970s and 1980s, particularly those who rejected the singular focus of feminists in the reproductive rights movement on abortion and contraception. Instead, they argued, a woman's right to *become* a mother (free of coercive state-sanctioned sterilization and racist contraception initiatives) was as important to a woman's "reproductive freedom" as the effort to liberate a woman from obligatory motherhood.[55] Religious and political commitments as pro-life activists have also put many homebirthers at odds with the broader rubric of reproductive rights. These women's commitment to natural childbirth became one more way in which they felt their concerns about reproduction and motherhood were ignored by feminists and reproductive rights activists. Instead, as one conservative midwifery supporter in Virginia explained to me, for her, telling legislators to "get out of our bedrooms" was a conservative sentiment, even though it allied with what she termed "radical feminist" aims.[56]

Sandelowski has gone so far as to suggest that the natural childbirth movement was actually "antifeminist": "It is simply inaccurate to politicize the early Natural Childbirth Movement. . . . In the 1940s and 1950s, there were no claims made to reproductive or other "rights" in relation to childbirth, unless it was the right to be happy. . . . Moreover, it was in line with the pronatalist sentiments of the times to keep women [particularly affluent white women] happy to have babies."[57] Perhaps the most accurate picture of natural childbirth proponents approximates what De Vries has described as "a motley crew— feminists, members of the religious right, 'back-to-the-earth' types, pro-family crusaders, peace activists, and libertarians   truly strange bedfellows."[58]

In the 1970s, the diversity of activists brought together by the natural childbirth movement began to be tested when emerging nationwide organizations included supporters from local, often like-minded support groups in a national dialogue about policy objectives. National groups, such as NAPSAC, attracted what historians Margot Edwards and Mary Waldorf have described in *Reclaiming Birth* as "a fiercely partisan and sometimes uneasy mixture of feminists determined to wrest from the male establishment women's rights to control their own reproduction, and traditionalists committed to preserving the integrity of the old self-reliant, self-contained American family."[59] Breastfeeding activists in the La Leche League and "traditionalist" and "maternalist" authors continued to focus in the 1960s and 1970s on "family-centered," unmedicated childbirth.[60] At the same time, feminists began to herald "woman-centered" childbirth, which fostered a woman's autonomy and strength, and diverse family relationships, which included women as friends and in collective communities,[61] mother-daughter bonds,[62] and lesbian relationships.[63] Similarly, differing attitudes about abortion divided many women in the natural childbirth movement between the "traditionalists," who supported a pro-life position, and the "feminists," who supported pro-choice politics.[64] The ideologies brought together in this movement were undeniably diverse but also representative of the shifting American values that influenced childbirth and reproductive healthcare activism in the twentieth century, "ranging from the cultural Left's critiques of the fragmentation of modern life and its separation from nature, to the feminist health movement's advocacy of medical self-help and women's right to reproductive choice, to the gender traditionalism and heteronormativity of breastfeeding advocates like the La Leche League, to religious fundamentalists' refusal of state intervention into the childbearing process."[65] Ultimately, the religious and political diversity of the natural childbirth movement became what anthropologist Karen Michaelson described as "an uneasy alliance of women who want[ed] similar birth experiences for very different reasons."[66]

Experiencing Natural Childbirth: Race, Class, and Cultural Difference

Despite this "uneasy alliance" of natural childbirth proponents, many middle-class white women created a public record of their struggle when they began to write about their own experiences of childbirth.[67] Their shared dissatisfaction with the medical management of reproduction in the United States united many otherwise politically and religiously diverse women. By the early 1970s, the combination of the largely successful activism within the natural childbirth movement and an emerging scholarly interest in reproduction stimulated a surge in hybrid scholarly-activist texts about childbirth. This literature drew together narratives of the authors' personal experiences in childbirth, cultural analyses of reproduction, support for women to resist medical norms in childbirth, and an enthusiastic push for women to engage in activism for access to childbirth alternatives.

Historical and sociological studies—designed for both scholarly and popular audiences—demonstrated the patriarchal origins of the medical management of childbirth and inspired many women to reevaluate their experiences of hospital birth.[68] Natural childbirth proponents also began to write their own instructional manuals, self-help handbooks, and guides regarding childbirth options.[69] Some of these books advocated unassisted childbirth, a birth option that became more widely discussed in the 1980s and 1990s,[70] and, more recently, through online forums dedicated to what many now call "freebirth," "DIY (do-it-yourself) birth" or "U-birth." Particularly in areas where midwifery has been illegal or unavailable, unassisted childbirth has offered women a legal alternative to hospital-based care, since homebirth itself is legal in all fifty states (only those who attend homebirths as practitioners are regulated). Taken together, these publications (and now online resources) have encouraged many women to envision childbirth not only as a personal event but also as an explicitly political issue.

Yet despite the personal becoming political for some women, others were losing access to the midwives who had traditionally practiced in their communities. Debra Susie, an anthropologist who conducted interviews with

remaining "granny midwives" in Florida in the 1980s as the "midwifery renaissance" was intensifying among middle-class white women,[71] wrote starkly:

> Birthing fads such as underwater childbirth, champagne breakfasts,
> and videotaped labors are not the only reasons that the new mid-
> wifery will never be the old midwifery. The latter evolved organically
> from a culture, while the former is a self-conscious acculturation. . . .
> Compromise with the state [regarding regulation and licensure] has led
> to the state's successful attainment of a long-awaited goal: the replace-
> ment of the traditional lay midwife with the modern nurse-midwife.[72]

Indeed, although African American midwives continued to serve marginalized women in the 1970s and 1980s in many areas of the United States, they
were invisible enough for the emerging profession of middle-class white midwives to describe itself as a "rebirth of midwifery."

Scholars of reproductive healthcare have further suggested that the singular
focus on "natural childbirth" in this more recent movement led many women to
romanticize the scope of "choice" in motherhood and childbirth.[73] For instance,
anthropologist Ellen Lazarus observed that while middle-class women indicated
control and choice as their top priorities in birthcare services, low-income
women responded to their more restricted options in childbirth with concerns
about continuity of care and being treated with respect by their practitioners.[74]
Moreover, a study by sociologist Margaret Nelson showed that women not only
had different *ideas* about what they wanted in childbirth, but they also had different experiences during the actual birth—working-class women's birth experiences were marked by less client participation and more medical intervention
than middle-class women's birth experiences.[75]

These studies have prompted a critical reassessment of natural childbirth
proponents' ideas about what was indeed "natural" for women in childbirth.
And, as anthropologist Margaret MacDonald has noted, "The portrayal of midwifery as an ancient tradition—timeless, enduring, universal—is closely related to the problematic notion of midwifery as an extension of women's *natural*
birthing and mothering experiences."[76] For example, in *Women Writing Childbirth*, literary scholar Tess Cosslett has criticized literature that advocated
"natural childbirth" as a return to the childbirth experiences of "primitive"
women.

> A powerful image in the natural childbirth-story has always been "the
> primitive woman": anyone who has been to antenatal classes will prob-
> ably recognize the stereotype. Often identified as "African," she goes

into the bushes on her own, gives birth painlessly and without fuss, and returns immediately to her work in the fields. . . . The primitive woman is, however, not nearly so primitive as she seems: she is a cultural construct, incorporating the maternal ideals of a particular society, and, paradoxically, her instinctive wisdom has to be learnt from books by "civilized" women.[77]

Suzanne Arms, for instance, a pioneer in the natural childbirth movement, provides a potent example of this idealized "story" about an unidentified "ancestral" culture in the introduction to her groundbreaking book *Immaculate Deception* in 1975:

> Imagine your distant ancestor in her late teens, living in a small village on the edge of a forest. She is a member of a small group of hunters and food gatherers. The time is late summer, when days are warm but nights chilly. This young woman is ready to give birth. She lives in a small hut with several members of her blood family.[78]

The story continues with an archetypal illustration of "primitive" childbirth, followed by a discussion of "reclamation," a return to traditional childbirth practices, such as labor and birth without drugs, nutrition and exercise during pregnancy, and midwife-assisted home birth.[79] Although Cosslett's critique was leveled at authors from the 1960s and 1970s, activists and childbirth educators have continued to rely on the "primitive" childbirth story as an example of ideal birth. For instance, in 1990, physician Judith Goldsmith described a universalized "normal tribal birth" in her book *Childbirth Wisdom*: "Like pregnancy, birth was not a time of stress or abrupt change in traditional cultures. Many women simply stopped at the side of the road on their way to or from the fields, gave birth, picked up their babies, and went on with their work."[80]

Similarly, natural childbirth advocate Marcie Macari begins her recent book *She Births* with a poem evoking her primal and ancient connections to African drummers and dancers.

> *The Women start beating a drum.*
> *I find their rhythm in my abdomen, and slowly move forward:*
> *One step—look at the face.*
> *Second step—focus on the eyes.*
> *Third step . . .*
> *I see the African dancers, rehearsing their steps as I walk my last few.*
> *I see the circle being set—the fire at the center, the food and festivities.*

> *This will be the stage for my welcoming into this elite group—*
> *This* Women of a Thousand Generations.
>   *my heart swells.*[81]

Macari's affinity for African women quickly becomes eclipsed, however, by the quotes she provides from "women around the world . . . about birth" that, as a whole, mirror U.S. middle-class white women's accounts of their experiences in hospitals and homebirths.[82] Although it is entirely possible that *some* women in indigenous cultures have had little difficulty giving birth, universalized stories such as the aforementioned evoke "images of the 'Noble Savage,' uncorrupted by civilization" and ultimately affirm beliefs about the superiority of women in Western cultures.[83]

Many scholars have critiqued this tendency toward romanticizing and universalizing the childbirth experiences of non-Western women as what anthropologist Shelley Romalis has called "more natural than our own."[84] Yet defining natural childbirth also brings attention to the uneven experiences of childbearing women within North America, particularly as these women are shaped by different levels of access to reproductive options. Nelson notes a problematic irony, that "those who are most interested in women defining for themselves the nature and meaning of childbirth are, perhaps, guilty of prescribing a perfect birth for all women, regardless of individual needs or motivations."[85] Similarly, Chris Bobel, in her sociological study of what she calls "natural mothering," notes the irony of the claims by her middle-class white participants that they had "free choice" about whether to homebirth, breastfeed, or stay at home with their children but that women who did not "follow their hearts" to make the same decisions could not be considered "good" mothers.[86]

It is within this circumscribed context for what is understood as "natural" in childbirth and motherhood that Helena Michie and Naomi Cahn identify the precarious position in which many women find themselves when they "fail" to achieve what they perceive as a natural childbirth (frequently by requesting pain medication or undergoing a Cesarean section).[87] Although childbirth is unquestionably regulated in the hospital,[88] medicalized control is not merely a "top-down" process. Women's surveillance of other women's childbirth experiences—in this case, natural childbirth—can shape and constrain the individual choices women make in childbirth in much the same way medicalized assumptions about childbirth can. It is also important to remember that "natural childbirth" has been defined not only by its proponents but also by those seeking to affirm the technological management of hospital childbirth. As philosopher Jana Sawicki has warned, "resistance" to dominant medical ideas about childbirth can easily be "neutralized" when these ideas are incorporated into the existing system of values around medicalized child-birth, such as "natural childbirth" classes in the hospital that prompt women to "expect and accept medical interventions such as fetal monitors, labor induction, forceps, pain medication, and even Caesarean sections."[89]

The neutralization of struggles against medicalization has also led to what many natural childbirth proponents have critiqued as the ever-expanding definition of natural childbirth. In the first edition of *In Labor*, Rothman described this "slippery slope" from childbirth in the home without medication or surgical interventions to "no surgical incision at the time of birth (episiotomy), whether or not the woman was conscious, to consciousness alone, even with an epidural or spinal anaesthetic."[90] Perhaps even more stunning to many contemporary proponents of natural childbirth is an experience I had when discussing the natural childbirth movement with my grandmother. She was excited to tell me about her experience with "natural childbirth" when my mother was born—a vaginal birth that she could not remember clearly because it occurred under twilight sleep.[91] Some authors have decided to abandon the term "natural childbirth" altogether. Unassisted childbirth proponent Hygeia Halfmoon favors "primal mothering" which, she argues, is "an invocation of what you [readers] already know,"[92] and Block prefers "normal childbirth."[93] Yet these modifications have similar pitfalls and limitations. What constitutes "primal" or "normal" in a process as personal and unique as childbirth? Are women still constrained by whether their childbirth experiences and options can live up to such definitions?

Ultimately, the malleable definitions—and experiences—of natural childbirth have extended beyond (but also at times recapitulated) the essentialized ideals of "primitive" childbirth presented earlier. Indeed, scholars have shown that what we perceive as "natural" or "normal" is indeed learned (and revised) within particular cultural contexts, "loaded" with the experiences, expectations, abilities, and opportunities afforded to each mother.[94] One such revision has occurred within the context of consumer efforts to support midwives, efforts that have highlighted the importance of women's choice and control through natural childbirth. MacDonald explains that this "modern" version of natural childbirth involves the promotion of "the primacy of informed choice as a principle and an act . . . midwifery provides the context to say that choice and knowledge count, and women come to count on it."[95] With this intensifying emphasis on choice and control in childbirth as key elements in natural childbirth, it becomes increasingly important to address the disparities in women's childbirth experiences and options to better understand the contemporary movement for midwifery in the United States.

Contemporary Support for Midwifery
and Homebirth

As discussed earlier in this chapter, the ebb of the natural childbirth movement's focus on improving women's experience in the hospital gave way to increasing interest in homebirth in the 1980s and 1990s among middle-class, primarily white, women. In contrast to the national acclaim of the natural childbirth movement, however, the "homebirth renaissance" developed primarily through local struggles to support homebirth and midwifery services, largely in response to state and medical restrictions on midwifery. The current legal situation of direct-entry midwives (DEMs), the primary attendants of homebirth, and the regulations governing their practices vary widely from state to state. For instance, prior to 2005, Virginia did not license DEMs, and it was illegal for unlicensed midwives to practice; Florida licenses DEMs who have completed three years of midwifery education to attend "normal births" autonomously; Arizona has a licensure program that requires mandatory education, certifying exams, and a formal arrangement for collaboration with a physician; and Mississippi permits "females" to engage in the practice of midwifery but neither registers nor licenses the individual (leaving them vulnerable to case-by-case prosecution, since there is no statutory definition of midwifery).[96]

The availability of midwifery services in many areas has also been limited by a variety of other factors, including doctors' refusal to supervise midwives in jurisdictions where physician supervision is mandated and the increasing price of midwifery services, as insurance and medical institutions have become attracted to "alternative childbirth" as a money-making venture.[97] Furthermore, court cases have taken on a regulatory function in many states where there are no clear-cut regulations for DEMs. As De Vries explains, "Midwives are free to practice until they attract the attention of medical professionals. If a client of a midwife comes to the attention of a physician and the physician believes something improper was done, then the law is invoked as a regulatory mechanism and courts become the area of regulation."[98] In 2008, the continued concern about court cases against midwives was the impetus for the Big Push for Midwives' slogan "Legislation, not Prosecution."

Throughout these struggles, midwives have found consistent allies among childbearing women. Activism for access to midwifery services has become common in many states and has been supported on a national level by Citizens for Midwifery (CfM) since 1996 and, more recently, by the Big Push for Midwives (since 2008) and the MAMA Campaign (since 2009). Following the development of CfM by several mothers who were involved in local midwifery support groups in Kentucky, Georgia, and Kansas,[99] CfM originally advertised itself as "the only national consumer-based group promoting the Midwives Model of Care" by providing education and guidance for effective grassroots organizing on the state level, specifically with regard to legislative lobbying.[100]

The political and religious diversity of the natural childbirth movement has also continued in the recent support of midwives and homebirth, remaining a point of pride and, in some cases, continued conflict. Notably, it remains common for organizations that promote homebirth and midwives to ban historically controversial topics—such as circumcision and abortion—from meetings, correspondence, and Listservs to keep participants motivated to mobilize around their common goal. These continued divisions have become motivation for midwifery supporters' to identify as "consumers"—a term, without the liberal connotations of "activist" or "feminist," that appeals to politically and religiously diverse organizers. Although women first began calling themselves consumers in childbirth-related groups during the 1960s, it was not until the 1990s that this became a self-conscious, strategic (and at times an uneasy) identity. As Klassen explains, "By focusing on consumer advocacy and choice and avoiding conflicts around sexuality and abortion, these allies formed a grass-roots, if fragile and loosely organized, 'alternative birth movement' that has had significant—although not always intended—effects both on trends in hospital care and on the visibility of home birth."[101]

Another related development has been the "consumer demand" for doulas, labor companions who provide women (and their families) emotional and physical support during and after labor.[102] Block has described the doula as a "distinctly American creation, arising out of a social deficit in maternity care [due to medicalization] and a consumer demand to fill it."[103] Most doulas are hired privately and paid for out of pocket,[104] though volunteer doula programs also exist throughout the United States that support low-income teenage women, recent immigrants, and incarcerated women.[105] What is interesting is that some hospitals have hired doulas specifically to meet women's increasing demand for personalized maternity care—not unlike the introduction of birthing suites and a more "homelike" environment during the 1970s, which assuaged some natural childbirth advocates but did not fundamentally change the medical management of labor in the hospital. Yet doulas have a voice, albeit frequently mediated by their tenuous position as nonmedical participants in many hospital births. Nevertheless, doulas' encouragement for women to "get what [they] want" out of childbirth is increasingly being heard by both birthing women and hospitals.[106]

Women's increased unification around "consumer rights" and "consumer choices" in healthcare regarding access to midwives, doulas, or even elective Cesareans has highlighted other issues of conflict among midwifery organizers, particularly regarding women's increasingly uneven access to healthcare at the turn of the twenty-first century. For example, during the 1980s, 30 percent of obstetricians stopped accepting Medicaid patients, primarily because of low reimbursement rates and concerns about medical malpractice liability.[107] New challenges have arisen for contemporary midwifery and homebirth advocates because of the rising numbers of uninsured among the middle class. As communications and rhetoric scholar Linda Miller explains in her analysis of legislative debates over midwifery in Florida:

> Birthing reform arguments which had centered on ideological choice [in the 1960s and 1970s], narrowed rapidly to consumer choice [in the 1980s and 1990s]. Moreover, arguments anchored in consumer choice increasingly became less relevant to middle class readers threatened with the prospect of joining the ranks of uninsured or underinsured "medical indigents." Instead of thinking about a range of birthing options, the focus shifted to what was affordable.[108]

As more luxury childbirth services have become available to affluent women, the options for poor women, uninsured women, and women on Medicaid have become further restricted. This broad stratification of access to healthcare resources has had mixed effects on efforts to gain access to midwives.

In one encouraging example of legislation that has improved access to midwives for a broad spectrum of women, Robbie Davis Floyd, Staccy Leigh Pigg, and Sheila Cosminsky tell the story of how middle-class white clients and contemporary homebirth midwives in Florida rallied around two black granny midwives, Gladys Milton and her daughter Maria.[109] When these granny midwives attended the births of primarily poor black women, they were largely ignored by the state healthcare system. However, when middle-class white women began seeking their services during the "midwifery renaissance" of the 1970s and 1980s, the state attempted to put them out of practice. Instead, the well-established clients and contemporary midwives who had organized, lobbied for legislation, and started their own midwifery schools, lobbied for the granny midwives. Ultimately, both contemporary DEMs and the two granny midwives gained licensure, "cementing what Florida midwives lovingly refer to as 'the alliance between the grannies and the granolas.'"[110]

In other states, however, the African American midwives who practiced throughout most of the twentieth century have not fared so well. For example, in her study of the elimination of African American midwifery in North Carolina, Holly Mathews emphasizes the fundamental shift in the priorities of those who have sought midwifery care over the past hundred years:

The central issue was reconceptualized . . . to be one of choice and
not access. . . . [Contemporary midwifery supporters in North Carolina had a] genuine desire to protect women's interests by preserving
the right to home birth in the face of strong challenges to it from the
medical community. . . . Yet in forging a compromise that restricted
such a right to women with access to registered nurse-midwives, [they]
sacrificed the interests of the numerically much larger group of poor,
rural, and predominantly nonwhite women who were left without access to care. . . . This happened in part because lay midwives had no
base of support from which to lobby during this campaign. The surviving elderly, black midwives located mainly in the rural eastern
counties were not involved at all in the political process, while the
young, urban white women desiring to practice lay midwifery were
perceived by many lawmakers to comprise a small fringe group of
"hippies" without credibility.[111]

Further, Gertrude Fraser found that the few African American midwives
who were still practicing in the United States in the 1980s usually attended
births for middle-class white women "who [were] able to choose freely, confident that they and their offspring [would] be afforded the best that midwifery
and science [had] to offer."[112]

The demographic statistics regarding homebirth also suggest a continued
racialized divide among those seeking homebirth and midwifery care. According to a study of U.S. homebirths as they were reported on birth certificates between 1989 and 1992, homebirthing women were primarily white,
and the health of their baby was likely to be better than that of the average
baby born in the United States.[113] While this study found that more white
women on the whole had homebirths, there was a stark racialized division in
the outcome of homebirths. White homebirthers tended to have more formal
education and better birth outcomes than other white women, while African
American homebirthers tended to have less formal education and poorer
birth outcomes than other African American women.[114]

In contrast, CNMs primarily attend hospital births for a variety of women.
As public health scholar Jennifer Parker explains:

Compared with all US births in 1988, for example, midwife-attended
hospital births (87% of all midwife-attended births) were more common among women who were non-White, younger, less educated, and
unmarried. The use of midwives for perinatal care has been found to
have no adverse effects on birth outcomes, in spite of the dominance

of women at higher risk for poor pregnancy outcomes among midwife patients.[115]

Parker further indicates that by the late-1980s, white mothers had begun to utilize midwives more frequently—with both CNMs and DEMs, in the home, in the birth center, and in the hospital.[116] Yet, the rates of midwife-attended births among African American, Hispanic, Native American, and Asian women, however, were decreasing, despite the positive birth outcomes associated with midwives.[117]

With the increasing commercialization of many "alternative healthcare" services, including midwifery,[118] this discrepancy further demonstrates how women of color continue to struggle harder to obtain good-quality, accessible healthcare than most of their Euro-American counterparts.[119] As Fraser explains, most middle-class African American women have divorced themselves from midwifery care, largely because of the successful dissemination of stereotypes associating midwives from their communities with poverty:

> I am convinced that the almost total success of the dominant ideology among African American women, especially among the middle class, came in large part because these women wanted to distance themselves from the pejorative racial stereotypes used to characterize the traditional midwife and those who depended on her skills. Going to the hospital or using a doctor at home became a marker of status among African American women. Ironically, the relatively inexpensive service of the midwife became less desirable because it was seen as an indication of poverty and "backwardness," and perhaps even as a measure of a woman's "insensibility" to the welfare of her unborn child.[120]

Similarly, historian Charlotte Borst has noted that immigrant mothers in the North also came to favor hospital birth at least in part because it distanced them from prejudices that they "clung to" outmoded ideas about childbirth.[121] As women of color and immigrant women internalized these prejudices, many came to see hospital birth as more desirable.[122] For immigrant women, hospital birth was also established as a distinctly American practice—one that contributed to their efforts to be seen as "good" American mothers.

Despite the marked differences in women's experiences of childbirth in the United States, the negative experiences many women have had (and continue to have) with medicalized childbirth, coupled with the restrictive government regulation of midwives, have generated new support for midwives in recent years. Community-based, statewide, and national organizations that support midwives have appeared and intensified throughout the country, continuing to draw women from a variety of religious, political and, increasingly, socioeconomic backgrounds who find it necessary to band together to ensure community access to homebirth midwives.

3

Midwives in Virginia

Educated, Eliminated, Criminalized,
and Rediscovered

While many . . . women root their choices [to homebirth] in
notions of a long-standing tradition of midwifery, most of
those views of tradition are not tied to distinct, living, or
directly remembered traditions with common cultural and
religious moorings.

—Pamela Klassen, *Blessed Events*

Although many scholars and activists have imagined a history of "sisters in struggle" for midwives over the past century, the poignant gap between predominately African American and immigrant women's support of midwives in the early 1900s and the "rebirth" of struggle for new forms of midwifery among primarily white women in the late twentieth century demonstrate quite different social and political milieus for both midwives and their supporters. In addition, the shifting racial and socioeconomic backgrounds of midwives and homebirthers in the United States have also had significant impacts on the results of their efforts. The virtual elimination of African American midwives during the twentieth century, for example, contrasts sharply with the recent successes of primarily white midwives and their supporters in the twenty-first century. Despite these differences, however, contemporary legislative debates over midwifery make it clear that some of the race- and class-based prejudices associated with the elimination of African American midwives still creep into contemporary public debates over midwifery licensure, as I explore in Chapter 4.

Thus this local history of midwives and their supporters in Virginia has a dual goal: to reveal the distinct differences in the experience of midwives in Virginia over the past one hundred years and to highlight the continued racial and class tensions evident in the long-standing medical, legal, and state opposition to midwives and homebirth.[1] These histories are printed side by side not in an effort to romanticize a unified history of struggle over the past century but, rather, to analyze how historical disparities can continue to impact efforts to support midwives today. Regarding the authenticity of this history, it is important to note that the materials on which I relied for its construction are inevitably incomplete. As I discuss later in this chapter, many of the public records regarding midwives who practiced in the early 1900s were destroyed by the state. Without such documents, I reconstruct these histories from existing scholarship on midwifery in Virginia and nearby states, editorials and reports published in public health and medical journals, newspaper articles, legislative documents, the personal narratives of Virginia midwives that are available through their memoirs, and my own participant-observation at judicial and legislative hearings and gatherings of midwifery supporters since 1999. I also rely, as anthropologist Gertrude Fraser has done, on the memories of those I interviewed,[2] and I am particularly grateful to those who sent me hard-to-find articles and resources from their personal archives.

Education or Elimination? The Midwifery "Problem" in the Early 1900s

Much like the plight of midwives throughout North America in the early twentieth century, Virginia midwives found themselves at the center of a public health effort to "educate" and eventually to eliminate nonmedical healthcare providers. By the early 1900s, Virginia state officials and physicians were in agreement that midwives—primarily African American "granny" midwives—were detrimental to medical progress and would eventually need to be eliminated throughout the state.[3] However, a question remained over whether to "educate" and supervise the practicing midwives who served communities where hospitals and physicians were not yet available,[4] or to eliminate, as one physician put it in 1925, the "great army of ignorant women now practicing midwifery in this country."[5] Ultimately, a combination of both approaches succeeded in eradicating most midwives in Virginia by the late 1900s, but government and medical efforts to license, regulate, and monitor midwives during the early 1900s left a peculiar legal and social situation for midwives into the twenty-first century.

Between 1910 and 1912, Walter Plecker, a physician, county registrar, and later state registrar of Vital Statistics in Virginia (from 1916 to 1946), instituted a pilot program to supervise midwives in a rural Virginia county. Plecker advised state officials that the limited number of physicians and hospitals available to rural, poor white women and African American women in both rural and urban areas made it impossible to completely eliminate midwives. Instead, a program to teach midwives "elementary safety rules" about childbirth allowed the licensure, and the subsequent supervision, of practicing midwives. Plecker also instituted a standardized birth registration form, requiring information about the child's sex, name, and date of birth and the parents' names, ages, occupations, marital status, and skin color, which would enable him to compare the work of physicians and midwives.[6]

Ultimately, however, the requirement that birth attendants record the names, marital status, and skin color of the infant's parents put midwives in a precarious regulatory position within the communities they served, particularly after the state passed legislation for the "preservation of racial integrity" in 1924, paralleling the height of the national eugenics movement. A series of "racial integrity laws" made interracial marriage illegal and supported the sterilization of those deemed "unfit" by the state.[7] Thus if midwives reported mixed-race children, then they incriminated members of the African American community and risked violent repercussions particularly upon African American men.[8] At the same time, a midwife's falsification of such information was a felony, punishable by a year in the state penitentiary. Consequently, many African American midwives quit their practices.

Further, Plecker—who had been instrumental in the passage of the Racial Integrity Acts—rescinded the classification "Indian" for ancestors of native-born Virginia Indians (Chickahominy, East Chickahominy, Mattaponi, Monacan, Nanesemond, Pamunkey, Rappahannock, and Upper Mattaponi). In 1943, Plecker issued a list of surnames belonging to these "mongrel" families that initiated the reissue of birth certificates, reclassifying American Indians from either "white" or "Indian" to "Negro."[9] Consequently, Virginia's American Indian midwives were also threatened with imprisonment for listing "Indian" as a racial classification on birth certificates for children in their communities.[10] As Fraser aptly summarized in her historical ethnography *African American Midwifery in the South*, laws regulating and supervising midwifery during the early part of the twentieth century, "inevitably mixed arguments about the need to reduce maternal and infant mortality and to improve health care with those confirming the importance of maintaining the racial and social order."[11]

Although Plecker's pilot program, as well as the 1918 legislation that required all Virginia midwives to obtain licenses from the Bureau of Vital Statistics, was ostensibly designed to monitor reproductive health and to create a more accurate record of vital statistics in the Commonwealth, regulations also discouraged many midwives from practicing because of increased surveillance, literacy requirements, and the bureaucratic structure of reporting births.[12] To obtain a midwifery permit from the Bureau of Vital Statistics after 1918, for example, the midwife had to register with the local registrar, attend classes in safety and hygiene, provide one or more letters of recommendation from local physicians who were familiar with her practice, agree to report all births within ten days to the local registrar, and promise to abide by the ten safety rules outlined in the "Midwife Manual" (provided by the Department of Health). Moreover, to maintain her permit, the midwife had moral and social obligations to the state:

(a) **MORAL**: A midwife should first of all be a conscientious woman. She should realize her responsibility to the mother and child and always remember that at every birth she has the lives of two people in her hands. She should be of cheerful disposition, patient, with a well balanced nervous system.

(b) **TRAINING**: She should realize that neither her training nor experience has fitted her to handle any case except a normal one. It is not only her duty, but the law requires her to call in a physician immediately when the conditions of labor are not absolutely normal. Even a doctor with his years of study and training frequently is unwilling to handle an abnormal case alone and calls in another physician to assist him.

(c) **HEALTH OF MIDWIFE**: It is very important that a midwife should be in good health. She should be free from disease, especially tuberculosis, syphilis, or any other that may be communicable. She should not attend a childbirth after attending an infected case or an acute disease without first having washed herself, including her hair, and put on fresh clean clothes.

(d) **CLEANLINESS**: A midwife should be exceedingly clean about her person, take frequent baths, keep her nails, hands, and hair clean, and change her clothes often. This is necessary because germs live in unclean things.[13]

Through the enforcement of such regulations, public health officials, physicians, and local registrars had the authority to deny or revoke midwives' permits if the midwives were deemed "unfit" to practice (for example, if they refused to fill out forms, if they utilized "unapproved" childbirth techniques or, we can presume, if they did not possess a "cheerful disposition"). A midwife risked a fine for practicing without a permit.[14] Ultimately, the federally sponsored public health programs and the increasingly stringent policing of midwives conducted by public health nurses led to the steady decline of midwifery in Virginia during the mid-1900s.

The elimination of midwives also had broader effects on the communities in which midwives served. For example, the written evaluations required for state-mandated midwifery permits encouraged older, often illiterate midwives to retire and favored young midwives, who were viewed by medical officials as being more compliant.[15] Over time, this increased surveillance and regulation of midwives eroded respect for elderly midwives within the communities they served.[16] Paralleling efforts to discredit midwives, physicians also began to blame African American mothers, not only their midwives, for the high maternal and infant mortality rates (as much as three times that of whites in some areas) in their communities, largely ignoring the economic impoverishment that most African Americans faced at the time.[17] As Fraser explains:

> [Medical investigators judged maternal and infant deaths as] the woman's "failure" to properly interpret and act on the physical "danger signals" of her body, or her negligence in not seeking out adequate prenatal care. Again, the flawed assumption held by investigators was that these were deliberate or avoidable actions on the part of women who "failed" to take advantage of readily available health resources. . . . Few African Americans had access to affordable medical care even after the passage of the Sheppard-Towner Act and the lobbying efforts of the Children's Bureau.[18]

Even when African American women and other women classified as "Negro" were admitted to segregated clinics, many were understandably fearful of the eugenic sterilization forced on many women of color at that time.[19]

While Virginia kept no official records of midwives at the turn of the twentieth century, medical officials suggested that thousands of midwives were serving various communities around Virginia prior to the widespread use of physician-attended hospital births. In 1928, one physician praised the local health departments, which had "done a splendid piece of work by reducing the number of midwives in the state from nine thousand very ignorant and dirty creatures to four thousand eight hundred and forty [by the 1920s], only one thousand two hundred and thirty-three of whom are really active."[20] These numbers continued to fall to approximately 1,000 in 1950 and 600 by the 1960s.[21] Although this decrease corresponds to national trends, as in many other states the transition reflected uneven developments among various constituencies of women.

Not surprisingly, early campaigns against homebirth and midwives were directed at the white women who could afford physicians' services; indeed, urban white women of all classes and rural, affluent and middle-class white women in Virginia were the first to choose physicians over midwives.[22] For these women, physicians and hospitals would alleviate pain in childbirth (through medication) and maintain an appropriately sanitary environment. As hospital birth became increasingly mainstream for white women, middle-class, urban African American women began to deliver in hospitals as physicians allowed,[23] however, primarily rural, poor, white and African American women continued to use midwives into the mid-1900s.[24] Even into the 1950s and 1960s, Claudine Curry Smith, the last African American lay midwife to practice in the lower Northern Neck of Virginia (near Chesapeake Bay), explained how the racial divide in healthcare continued:

> Most of the White people had their doctors come to the house—they had the money to pay the doctor. Black people just didn't have the doctor's money. Midwives were cheaper. Insurance didn't cover having a midwife come. So, they'd pay out of their pocket. I delivered some white too, but the ones that did it said they'd rather have a midwife than go to the hospital.[25]

During the 1950s, health departments also began to require pregnant women to get an authorization card from a physician to approve a midwife-assisted delivery; these new requirements began to limit poor women's access to midwives because of the mandatory cost (and social pressures) of one or more prenatal doctor's visits.[26] As one physician summarized in 1966, "The old-fashioned uneducated midwife is fast disappearing, prenatal clinics have educated the poor who once employed them, and the ease of getting to a hospital where an intern or staff doctor will deliver them has eliminated the granny almost completely in many areas where she was popular even a decade ago."[27] Smith, who had practiced as a lay midwife for thirty-one years in the Northern Neck, explained how this shift was also impacted by physicians' financial interests:

> The doctors stopped coming to cover for the midwives, for mothers to be delivered at home, in those last ten years I practiced [the 1970s]. I don't know why. I've never known the reason, but they stopped coming to midwives. . . . But I think the doctors here was still supportive with the midwives. But see, the thing of it is that a lot of people wasn't able to pay the money the doctors were charging and if the midwives could do it, they were still the family doctors, so I think they didn't mind having a midwife.[28]

Nevertheless, Virginia's confidence in the progress of medically managed childbirth prompted the General Assembly's 1962 decision to move the regulation of midwives to the Virginia Department of Health (VDH) in an attempt to further limit midwifery practice to "rural, underserved areas, minority women, and poor, uninsured women."[29] The VDH granted midwifery permits to individuals who presented two letters of reference from practicing physicians, who observed and assisted with ten or more hospital deliveries, who passed an examination, and who conformed "with acceptable moral reputation and adhere[d] to high standards for personal cleanliness, neatness and demeanor."[30] Shortly after this transition, in 1965 the federal introduction of Medicaid reimbursement for deliveries performed by physicians, coupled with the Civil Rights Act of 1964, which officially ended the segregation of childbirth clinics, opened doors for poor women and women of color to access healthcare in the hospital and ultimately eliminated the need for midwives in many areas.[31] Following these developments, few records of the practices of midwives exist, either at local health departments or at the central offices of the VDH in Richmond. As nursing professor Mildred Roberson writes in *My Bag Was Always Packed*:

> In the Virginia Department of Health central offices in Richmond, the repository for what few records remain of midwives and their history, there is simply a folder containing a smattering of names of midwives in practice in selected counties, in specified years. Most records have been lost or destroyed. It is apparent that no one has maintained records in the central VDH office in Richmond on an ongoing basis. Staff now in the county health departments say that all required records were sent to Richmond, and all local records were destroyed for lack of space. The story is the same elsewhere in the South. As Debra Anne Susie commented in her book about Florida midwives: "The American midwife's misfortune was to lose not only her vocation but her history as well."[32]

Criminalizing "Lay Midwifery" in Virginia

In 1974, the VDH restricted applications for a midwife permit to "registered nurse[s] in good standing [who had graduated from] a school of midwifery accredited by the American College of Nurse Midwifery [*sic*]."[33] And, in 1976, the General Assembly enacted legislation that limited the practice of non-nurse midwifery to those who had received permits from the VDH prior to January 1, 1977. In effect, only the non-nurse midwives who had received permits prior to the change in regulations in 1974 were "grandmothered" in and allowed to continue to practice. After 1977, a family in Virginia remained legally entitled to homebirth with whomever they chose, though it became illegal for a midwife who was not previously permitted or registered as a nurse-midwife to practice. The Code of Virginia defined a midwife as "any person who, for compensation, assists in delivery and postnatal care by affirmative act or conduct immediately prior and subsequent to the labor attendant to childbirth in conjunction with or in lieu of a member of the medical profession."[34] Thus a non-nurse midwife who wished to be paid for her services was practicing outside of the law.[35] The law also made it illegal for a non-nurse midwife to receive any "gifts" as payment; "'Compensation' means anything of value received before or after the labor attendant to childbirth, with or without an express agreement between the person so assisting and the patient or anyone in the patient's behalf."[36]

The "success" of this legislation was well documented by the VDH. The number of lay midwives who had permits in Virginia hovered around one hundred in the 1980s and slowly decreased to just five in 1999.[37] Of the five midwives who had permits in 1999, one was living out of state, three were retired,[38] and the one lay midwife who practiced in Virginia until 2001 has since retired and moved out of the state.[39] Taken together, these legislative decisions had significant implications regarding who was able to practice (and access) midwifery in Virginia.

To replace lay midwives, the 1976 legislation introduced the licensure of the nurse-midwives as CNMs. Following the demographic trend among public health nurses who were tasked with "training" African American midwives in the early 1900s, most of the new nurse-midwives were white women who had the means to attend both nursing school and to complete a master's degree in nurse-midwifery. Even with master's level training—and unlike the regulations for CNMs in most other states[40]—the Virginia legislature did not allow the emerging profession to practice autonomously but, rather, only under a physician's supervision. In a practical sense, this meant that CNMs were required to have orders from a physician to administer all medical procedures and to conduct "their usual professional activities which shall include the taking of blood, the giving of intravenous infusions and intravenous injections, and the insertion of tubes."[41] This requirement made CNMs available only in areas where a local physician was willing to supervise their practice, which varied considerably throughout the state. A survey conducted by the Task Force on the Study of Obstetric Access and Certified Nurse-Midwives in 1992 found that overt resistance to CNMs was common among Virginia physicians:

> More than one-half [of CNM respondents] indicated that a physician had at least once tried to exclude them from providing care in their role as a nurse-midwife, and more than one-third had been exposed to a physician who refused to refer patients to them. More seriously in terms of public protection, nearly one-third reported that physicians

had refused to accept patient referrals from the nurse-midwife. These rejections ostensibly include high risk cases which are inappropriate for CNM care.[42]

One physician, citing the high malpractice risks associated with supervising a CNM, told a newspaper reporter in 1990 that he would "run in the other direction" if a CNM approached him about collaborating.[43] According to participants in my ethnographic research, in the late 1990s, CNMs had to close practices or were unable to practice in Richmond, Charlottesville, northwestern Virginia, and the Tidewater area because local physicians were not willing to supervise their birth center, homebirth, or even hospital practice.

Nevertheless, CNMs in Virginia increased from approximately eighty practitioners in the early 1990s to over 126 in 2000.[44] By the early 1990s, most of these CNMs practiced in hospital clinics that provided care for primarily indigent patients,[45] however, since that time, middle-class and affluent patients began to demand access to CNMs in hospitals, birth centers, and homes. Thus by the late 1990s, CNMs had begun to practice in more urban and suburban areas.[46] According to the most recent statistics from the American College of Nurse-Midwives, in 2008, 226 CNMs were licensed in Virginia and, in 2004, they attended 8.4 percent of Virginia births.[47] Although BirthCare and Women's Health, a nationally acclaimed birth center and homebirth practice run by CNMs, exists in northern Virginia, the number of CNM-run birth centers and home-based practices in operation has, in general, declined since the 1990s.[48] For example, the CNM-run birth center in Charlottesville closed in the late 1990s because it could no longer secure physician supervision for its practice, as midwifery supporter Ellen Hamblet explained in a presentation to the Board of Medicine, "abruptly leaving an entire community without the access they had come to rely on."[49] Other CNMs have not been able to find jobs practicing midwifery: the Task Force on the Study of Obstetric Access and Certified Nurse-Midwives indicated that at least one-third of Virginia CNMs were practicing outside of their chosen profession in 1991.[50] Moreover, five of the eight CNMs I interviewed in 2000 and 2001 were working outside of their field.

Although it is difficult to obtain accurate statistics on births with unlicensed midwives, because homebirth families frequently chose not to report the attendants at their births to protect midwives from state investigations, the Joint Commission on Health Care noted the increase in the number of births attended by "other midwives" between the 1980s and the 1990s—from a low of 35 in 1985, to 155 in 1995, to 303 in 1997, and to 500 births in 2000.[51] Yet the Joint Commission also acknowledged that the actual number of deliveries by direct entry midwives may be higher, as it is possible that some of the deliveries in the "other attendant" or "unknown" category were delivered by direct entry midwives. Clearly, the current legal status of direct entry midwifery creates a disincentive for a family in registering a birth to highlight that the birth was attended by a direct entry midwife.[52]

"Rediscovering" Midwifery: Homebirthers…and State Investigators

Virginia's "midwifery renaissance" echoed the national resurgence of interest in homebirth in the 1980s, prompting both CNMs and underground DEMs to offer homebirth services to a growing number of middle-class white families in many urban areas of Virginia. One newspaper article in 1990 contrasted homebirth CNMs to the granny midwives of years past:

> Modern training colors ancient role
> Midwives Alice Bailis and Marsha Jackson don't fit the image of the granny delivering babies in a mountain shack. Their combination of medical training and supportive care make them a popular choice for couples who want to play a more active role in the birth of their children.[53]

Alice Bailis and Marsha Jackson are the CNMs who established BirthCare and Women's Health in 1987 to provide homebirths in northern Virginia and in the Washington, D.C., metropolitan area (including areas of Maryland), and in 1992, they opened a freestanding birth center.[54] Other CNM practices in the D.C. area, such as the Maternity Center in Bethesda, Maryland, phased out homebirth practices during the late 1980s and early 1990s and have since closed. In contrast, BirthCare was committed to keeping homebirth available to women in the area, and the growing interest in homebirth allowed them to expand to a group of five CNMs, who continue to attend eighteen to twenty-five births a month, approximately 70 percent in clients' homes and 30 percent in their birth center.[55]

Also during the 1980s a handful of other CNMs—as well as a few doctors and osteopathic physicians—were providing homebirth services in Virginia, particularly in rural areas. Attesting to the continued socioeconomic diversity of Virginia's homebirth community, Juliana van Olphen-Fehr, a rurally based CNM who operated a homebirth service from 1984 to 1997 in northwestern Virginia, recalls in her published diary one of the "lessons" she learned from her clients:

> One of my first lessons was that many people who called for my services did not necessarily subscribe to the philosophy of the home birth movement. I learned quickly that just as not all midwives are alike, not all people who choose home birth are alike. Not all of the people who called wanted the privacy, the dignity and the "naturalness" that come with having a baby at home. A lot of people called me because they didn't have insurance and they couldn't afford the doctor or the hospital.[56]

During the 1980s and into the early 1990s, many unlicensed midwives felt safe continuing their homebirth practices, despite Virginia laws that had made their occupation illegal since the 1970s. For example, Sherry Willis, who offered homebirth services in the Blue Ridge Mountains of northern Virginia, told a reporter in 1990 that she preferred "the autonomy of her form of midwifery" to that of physician-supervised nurse-midwifery.[57] The reporter explained:

> She has never been sued, and, she says, has no fear of legal repercussions. No baby has ever died in her care.
>   "I'm a community-created midwife," she says. "I don't advertise. I didn't even have business cards for 10 years. These families have gotten to a point where they are emotionally and physically ready, and willing to accept the realities of nature."[58]

Similarly, Carol Cahours, an unlicensed midwife who practiced in central Virginia during the 1990s, told a reporter, "Everyone knows I'm here." Ironically, the 1996 article was entitled "Unlicensed Midwives Can't Practice Legally under Virginia Statute."[59]

While many unlicensed midwives disregarded the laws that were designed to eliminate their practice, others questioned their legal application. Stacy Newby, who had practiced legally as a "lay midwife" in Texas and California but had switched to offering birthing talks and facilitating childbirth support groups when she moved to the Northern Neck of Virginia, explained to a reporter in 1995:

> "Present Virginia laws define midwifery as being present at the time of birth and receiving payment for this. Payment could be anything: a goat, a painting, money, even just a thank-you. A licensed nurse midwife

may only facilitate labor and birth under the direct supervision of a physician. Obviously, the definitions of midwifery are a bit unclarified here. What if you suggested that a laboring woman drink a cup of tea or take a walk? What if you took her blood pressure for her at her request? Is this practicing midwifery or medicine?"[60]

During the mid-to-late 1990s—ironically, during the same period the aforementioned articles were being written—the state began to answer these questions by intensifying its investigations, and in several cases the criminal prosecution, of underground midwives and those who assisted them. For example, in 1994, Dr. Susan Osbourne had her license put on probation after providing backup services and ordering tests for an unlicensed midwife in Richmond, and was ordered to take fifty hours of obstetrical training.[61] For unlicensed midwives, however, the results of investigations were often more damaging. Martha Hughes, for example, who was nationally credentialed as a CPM (prior to CPMs' licensure in Virginia in 2005), stopped practicing after her arrest in a manslaughter case regarding a baby who died after a homebirth she assisted in 1995. The charges were eventually dropped because the baby's parents maintained that the midwife had done all she could to save their baby, and they refused to cooperate with the prosecution.[62] Following her arrest, Hughes, after attending over two hundred births in Virginia, became a part-time waitress in Rappahannock County.[63] Because of Hughes's early retirement, several former and potential clients were not able to have homebirths because they could not find local practitioners.[64] The fear surrounding these increased investigations and legal cases became an effective tool for the state to discourage other midwives from providing homebirths.

As a case in point, during a highly publicized criminal case against another midwife in Virginia, both the state prosecutor and the judge felt it important not only to put the midwife involved on trial but also to send a "clear message" to "deter others who are similarly situated."[65] In 1999, Cynthia Caillagh, a widely known DEM who had attended approximately 2,500 homebirths during her career as a midwife in New York, Tennessee, and Virginia, and her assistant, Elizabeth Haw, were charged with involuntary manslaughter, practicing midwifery without a license, and practicing medicine without a license after their client, Julia Peters, died following a homebirth in 1997. The medical examiner's report cited postpartum hemorrhage as the cause of death, but Caillagh and Haw's attorneys, as well as their supporters, maintained that the cause of Peters's death was open to question. Before the trial, supporters suggested in a press release that the lab report documenting Peters's hemoglobin and hematocrit levels—9.8 and 22, respectively—did not support the diagnosis of postpartum hemorrhage,[66] and that the delayed issuance of the medical examiner's report—eight months after the date of death—was significant to the defense's case.[67]

Nearly three years after Peters's death, one of the first events I attended with homebirthers in Virginia was the plea bargain hearing that brought Caillaigh's trial to an end in 2000. Over one hundred supporters came from all over Virginia. Apart from the impressive number of women who gathered there, many sitting on colorful blankets and playing with their children on the courthouse lawn, I was also struck by the racial diversity of the families that attended. All of the legislative hearings I would later attend with midwifery supporters drew primarily white midwives and mothers, but Caillagh's practice clearly drew a wider group of homebirthers. When I later asked one of Caillagh's clients—who identified herself and her children as "mixed," with a family heritage including American Indian (Cherokee ancestry she shared with Caillagh), English, Scottish, Welsh, French, Filipino, Chinese, Portuguese, and Spanish—about her experience attending legislative hearings with her children, she replied glibly, "It's definitely too lily-white for me. I mean, shoot, any time we show up my kids are the token color, you know." Most other women of color opted out of attending legislative proceedings, but as one of Caillagh's African American clients later explained, attending public events associated with the trial was different for her, because "I wanted the best for Cynthia. I didn't want her to go to jail. . . . When you called me, I was in tears when you called me [to ask for an interview], the bond was so strong. She's like a part of the family."

Unlike legislative hearings, children were not allowed in the courtroom, so small groups of women remained outside to allow other mothers to enter. The courtroom itself was packed, both with reporters and Caillagh's supporters. As a result, security was tight, and at one point, a deputy inspected the notebook in which I was writing to ensure that I was not audiotaping the hearing. The prosecution had already chosen to drop the manslaughter charge—which would have required a full trial—in part because of the publicity of defense attorney Peter Greenspun's case,[68] which involved using expert witnesses to testify against the medical examiner's report,[69] and in part because Daren Peters, Julia Peters's husband, maintained that the midwives "did their job," and thus he refused to cooperate with prosecutors.[70] Amid the tears and heavy sighs of her supporters, Caillagh pleaded guilty to practicing midwifery without a license, practicing medicine without a license (based on testimony regarding her use of Pitocin and her performance of an internal vaginal exam),[71] and neglecting an incapacitated adult. Haw pled guilty to practicing midwifery without a license. Both received suspended jail sentences, were fined $2,500 and $500, respectively, and promised to stop delivering babies unless the state law was changed. In a press release following the trial, Caillagh indicated that the prosecution's agreement to drop charges against Julia Peters's mother-in-law,

Claire Peters,[72] and to reduce charges against Haw weighed heavily in her decision to plead guilty to the three misdemeanors.[73]

The national impact of this case continued because the case not only received extensive media coverage but was covered in Jennifer Block's 2007 book on midwifery, *Pushed!* [74] Even more broadly, however, under U.S. law the case had wider implications for pregnant women. The final charge against the midwife in this case, her violation of a statute governing care provided to incapacitated persons, is most commonly brought to bear in cases intended to protect patients in mental institutions and nursing homes, those who are unable to consent to treatment and who have no authorized person to consent to treatment on their behalf.[75] This sets a disturbing precedent. Based on Virginia case law, the definition of an "incapacitated person" now includes a pregnant woman in labor, and her husband's consent for treatment was determined insufficient by the Caillagh case. As political scientist Rachel Roth has demonstrated in her broader work on the legal coercion of pregnant women (through court-ordered Cesarean sections, for example), physicians and judges are increasingly defining mentally competent pregnant women as "irrational, incompetent, and bad,"[76] a concern I explore in greater detail in Chapter 4.

Another reason this case garnered broad media attention both locally and nationally was because it coincided with the introduction of legislation to decriminalize the practice of DEMs in Virginia. This publicity was both positive and negative. A prominent five-part series of articles in 1998 in Fredericksburg's newspaper, *The Free Lance-Star*, drew critical attention to Peters's death and the legal controversy surrounding it.[77] The battery of letters to the editor from Caillagh's and Haw's supporters, however, suggested a distinct bias in reporting and began to refer to the investigation as a "witchhunt," a "bogus investigation," and a "political persecution" of alternative healthcare practitioners in Virginia.[78] In response, Stafford Circuit Judge James Haley Jr. turned directly to Callaigh's and Haw's many supporters who were seated in the courtroom during their plea bargain to declare, "This prosecution was not a persecution," and he repeated the statement twice more for effect.[79] Subsequently, the prosecuting attorney, Eric Oleson, told a reporter that Caillagh's guilty pleas "prohibit her from being a martyr."[80]

Other reporters cited connections between the investigation and the legislation that midwifery supporters were introducing to the General Assembly in 1999 to decriminalize the practice of DEMs in Virginia:

> Now, debate about state regulation of childbirth has been reborn. Two midwives were charged with manslaughter in January in the case of a Stafford County woman who died after her baby was born at home in 1997.

Such rare criminal cases have inspired media onslaughts, but the intense publicity may do little to clear up myths about traditional midwifery. Virginia's 22-year-old ban on the practice probably has compounded the mysteries by forcing practitioners to operate without detection.[81]

Marsden Wagner, a well-known physician who supports midwifery and the former director of the Women's and Children's Health Program in the European Office of the World Health Organization, wrote in an editorial for *The Roanoke Times*:

It can be no accident that these midwives have been charged just at the moment the Virginia General Assembly is considering new legislation on midwifery. But health care in Virginia should be determined on the basis of the best scientific evidence and not on the basis of unproven, anecdotal horror stories.[82]

Following the case, Caillagh moved out of state, and Haw abandoned her plan to become a midwife. After the trial, supporters continued to rally around Caillagh and Haw, as many shifted their attention to legislation to decriminalize the practice of DEMs in Virginia. Reaffirming many homebirthers' concerns for their midwives, Debbie Goodman wrote for the Voices for Healthcare Rights Fund's "Trial Update" in 2000:

During the past 2-½ years the Stafford County courts and the media have made Julie [Julia Peters] into a naïve victim. The charge of Neglect of an Incapacitated Adult is an insult to Julie, Daren, Cynthia, and to every woman who has ever given birth. The trial in Stafford may be over, but its wounds will be felt for a very long time. All of us who support a family's right to informed decision-making in all areas of our lives need to work together to change the laws in Virginia and stand in defense of one another and our practitioners. Don't let this happen to another midwife or another family again.[83]

Emerging Activism for Virginia Midwives among Homebirth Mothers

In light of the increased state investigation of midwives during the 1990s, midwives became further limited in their ability to engage in public advocacy for their profession, and many closed their homebirth practices. By the end of the 1990s, CNMs offered homebirth services only in the areas surrounding Richmond and northern Virginia.[84] In 1998, the VDH estimated that twenty to thirty underground midwives were practicing throughout the state, though "this number is impossible to verify empirically and . . . may be too high."[85] Furthermore, many of these practitioners had also begun to restrict their clients to women they knew personally or through other trusted sources. Thus it was the decreasing availability of homebirth as midwives were forced to close their practices that became the catalyst for grassroots organizing among homebirth mothers. This support for midwifery in Virginia initially came from local groups that were often centered around a midwife or a handful of midwives serving their communities.

For instance, Peninsula Families for Natural Birth and Health Care (Pen-Fam) was founded in the Virginia Beach area in 1996 by "five moms wishing to create a support network for clients of our local direct-entry midwife as well as provide information for the general public about natural birth and health care."[86] PenFam eventually dissolved, and two organizations emerged in the Virginia Beach area, each pursuing one of PenFam's stated goals: Families for Natural Living (FNL) remains active as an educational organization for "informed healthcare" decisions, and Voices for Healthcare Rights Fund (Voices), which began officially in 1998 but is no longer active, focused primarily on generating financial and organizational support for the defense of local midwife Caillagh and her assistant Haw.

Shortly after the formation of PenFam in Virginia Beach, Steve Cochran organized Virginia Birthing Freedom (VBF) in southwestern Virginia. In 1997, VBF, represented by a professional lobbyist, brought the issue of increased public interest in DEMs to the attention of the General Assembly during the public commentary period of a state study to improve access to prenatal care and childbirth facilities in rural and underserved areas, the Perinatal/Early Childhood Subcommittee of the Maternal and Child Health Council. This prompted a successful resolution for the Joint Commission on Health Care (JCHC) to initiate a midwifery study in 1998 to examine "the advisability of legalizing direct-entry midwifery," with assistance from the Department of Health Professions and the Department of Health,[87] which I discuss further in Chapter 4.[88] Between 1998 and 2001, a proliferation of other groups formed throughout the state to support midwifery, including Harrisonburg Advocates for the Midwifery Model of Care (HAMMOC), Richmond Families for Birthing Alternatives (RFBA), Fredericksburg Area Consumers of Homebirth and Midwifery Care, Mothers United for Midwifery (MUM), in the Roanoke area, and Midwifery Options for Mothers (MOM), in northern Virginia. One of the issues that divided many of these groups was whether midwives should be supported by pushing for licensure (and thus, potentially restrictive regulation by the state), or DEMs' practices should be decriminalized (which would allow practitioners to regulate themselves, however, they would remain vulnerable to charges of practicing medicine or nurse-midwifery without a license).[89]

One organization, in 1999, attempted to unite these groups in the Virginia Midwifery Coalition (VMC) by promoting a "unity of purpose" among Virginia midwifery groups. An e-mail invitation to join the coalition from organizer Brynne Potter read as follows:

> What we are severely lacking are communication and trust between the various groups in Virginia who seem to have the same goals. That common goal as I see it is to promote greater access to direct entry midwifery. . . . We are also in agreement that an arching coalition/ council would be a multi-faceted benefit to each groups' [sic] existing agenda because of the obvious networking that would come out of communicating better. We each in varying degree[s] understand that we all need each other to reach our goals. . . . I think this is a labor, and we are in transition. If we are going to deliver safely, we need to join hands and learn to trust each other.[90]

While the VMC itself was short-lived, attempts to unify groups supporting midwifery continued in Virginia. In particular, the advent of the JCHC midwifery study in the late 1990s renewed organizers' efforts to mobilize midwifery supporters by maintaining mailing lists of midwives' clients and other supporters and developing statewide Listservs to connect advocates.

Two professional organizations for midwives also provided support during this time. The Commonwealth Midwives Alliance (CMA) was formed in 1983 to support midwives who sought "full access to legal, autonomous midwifery services, in all setting[s], for the citizens of Virginia."[91] CMA served as a consistent support network for DEMs and became a major player in the passage of legislation to legalize CPMs in 2005, after the law prohibiting DEMs was struck down in 2003, allowing midwives to become more visible in political struggles. I return to these legislative developments in more detail in Chapter 4. The second professional organization for midwives was the Virginia Chapter of the American College of Nurse-Midwives (VACNM), which was formed in 1984. Virginia's chapter of ACNM is the primary organizing body for all nurse-midwives. Although most CNMs practice in the hospital, several VACNM members continue to work on legislation to improve CNMs' ability to provide homebirth in Virginia. In 1999, VACNM also officially supported efforts to legalize CPMs in Virginia, in addition to the ACNM-based certification credential for non-nurse midwives, the CM.[92] This initial support was a notable break from the national ACNM policy of opposing the licensure of any midwives who were not certified by their organization. In recent years, many individual CNMs have maintained their support of legislation that benefits CPMs, but VACNM did not offer its official support for legislation to license CPMs (which was successful in 2005). When I asked CNMs who participated in my study about this shift, most highlighted Virginia CNMs' tenuous relationship with individual physicians and medical organizations in the state, and they expressed concerns over reprisal by the physicians who supervise them (and therefore determine whether or not they are able to practice). Some CNMs had received letters or verbal warnings from physicians— saying that if Virginia's chapter of ACNM supported CPM legislation, then prominent medical associations would withhold their support from future legislation to benefit CNMs. These unsteady alliances—and the fears of state and medical repercussions that underlie the political decisions of all midwives—serve as a potent reminder of the hostile climate that continues to impact the history of midwifery in Virginia.

Reviewing the events that eliminated one form of midwifery and led to the rediscovery of others during the past century in Virginia, it becomes clear that emerging activism among homebirth mothers is part of a legacy with a complicated past. At present, there is little personal memory of African American midwives among contemporary organizers in Virginia, though most midwifery supporters are well versed in the history of medical opposition to midwifery since the early 1900s. Although some are tempted to articulate these events as a seamless and unified history, to do so glosses over the important differences in midwives'—and mothers'—distinct histories and experiences. These histories do share some common ground, however, through the disrespect and hostility that midwives and the mothers who support them still face from state and medical officials. This, in some cases, unearths the racial and socioeconomic tensions of earlier eras as it continues to punctuate today's struggles for midwives.

4

Mothers in the Legislature

Claiming Respectable
American Motherhood

"Reproductive politics" in the twenty-first century is a
struggle between women claiming the right to make
decisions about their own lives and their own bodies,
against an increasingly demanding, intrusive central
government that more and more frequently invokes religious
and corporate language to justify power over women's
bodies and their lives.
——RICKIE SOLINGER, *PREGNANCY AND POWER*

S ince medical licensing campaigns gained governmental support in the
early 1900s, challenges and alternatives to the medical management of
childbirth have fallen under the scrutiny and control of local and federal
lawmakers.[1] Because professional licensure is handled at the state level in the
United States, debates over the regulation of midwives have occurred in state
legislatures throughout the nation since the early 1900s. Published accounts
of these debates—both historically and during the past few decades—suggest
that the assessment of "good" and "bad" midwives has been a primary concern in efforts to license midwives.[2] In the Virginia legislature, however, politically active mothers bore the brunt of medical officials' attacks against
midwifery and homebirth. Both medical and state officials evoked the image
of "bad mothers" and even their "bad babies" to make a case against homebirth and midwives instead of (and sometimes in addition to) the familiar
stereotypes about "bad midwives."

Thus homebirth mothers' decision to lobby for midwives in legislative
debates created the need for a new kind of midwifery advocate—one who
supported midwives from her position as a respectable American mother, not
as a midwife herself. Just as midwives have responded to the need to become
"ambassadors of the profession" in other legislative struggles,[3] homebirth
mothers in Virginia also found themselves "disciplined" by the state regarding

respectable American motherhood. As women's bodies have historically been subject to social control within medical institutions, they have been similarly under surveillance by the government, which serves as the ultimate authority over who is and who is not considered a legitimate mother (that is, a mother who is legally entitled to make choices for herself and her children).[4]

Yet as social theorist Michel Foucault has demonstrated, the "power of the norm" functions not only through direct surveillance by those in power but also in the ways that the surveillance is intensified when members of society keep watch over one another and themselves.[5] Within this context, homebirth mothers advocating for midwives worked hard to present themselves—and other homebirthers—as good American mothers, despite their unconventional decision to birth in the home. Most women, at the turn of the twenty-first century, achieved respectable mother status (at least in part) by giving birth in the hospital. Anthropologist Robbie Davis-Floyd has described the process of birth in obstetrical settings as an American rite of passage that "transform[s] the birthing woman into a mother in the full social sense of the word—that is, into a woman who has internalized the core values of American society."[6] As we have seen in previous chapters, ideals and expectations about what has constituted good (and bad) motherhood have shifted over time. It was during the legislative debates over midwifery in Virginia at the turn of the twenty-first century that many midwifery advocates began to forge a new identity as midwifery consumers who could make educated, responsible choices about where and with whom to have their babies.

Legislative Efforts for Midwives in Virginia: 1998–2002

I attended my first legislative hearing regarding midwifery legislation in Virginia's General Assembly in 1999. I sat with a small group of midwives and homebirth mothers who had traveled to Richmond from throughout the state (several women had woken up at 3 A.M. to be there for the early-morning meeting). Many of their children played quietly on the floor, and several mothers sat in small, folding chairs awkwardly breastfeeding their newborns and toddlers. Most homebirth mothers viewed their efforts to bring their children to the legislature as evidence of their "good" mothering practices—they were mothers who would not leave their children at home with a babysitter so that they could pursue their own interests.[7] A handful of legislators sat in front of us on cushioned desk chairs behind heavy wooden tables, waiting for the hearing to begin. Their desks were positioned in several semi-circles on ascending risers so that they literally looked down on those who were gathered to listen to the proceedings. A low podium was positioned on the floor in front of the audience, where speakers would stand to address the legislators.

I realized as I sat in the audience that not only was this my first experience attending a legislative hearing on midwifery, but it was also the first time I had ever been in a legislative building. Having grown up largely outside of the United States, I thought initially that I would be alone in my naïveté about American politics. But as several homebirthers explained to me before the hearing began, few of the women that attended in support of their midwives had ever participated in U.S. politics in this way. In fact, one young mother broke the awkward silence of the half-filled hearing room when she laughingly admitted to watching Schoolhouse Rock's "How a Bill Becomes a Law" the night before, more for her own benefit than for her children's. As we collectively reviewed the political process, another mother recited a portion of the Gettysburg Address with her homeschooled children, that American politics is a "government of the people, by the people, for the people."[8] In contrast to this impromptu lesson in democratic governance, when I glanced at the legislators who were now getting ready to convene the meeting, I found myself troubled by how distanced and distracted they appeared. Clearly uncomfortable with the presence of mothers and children—perhaps especially the mother who was now nursing in the front row—they averted their eyes from their audience, choosing instead to fiddle with computers, to rustle paperwork, and to read newspapers. This continued as the presenters were called to approach the podium. Ultimately, the speakers' well-rehearsed presentations of research on the safety of homebirth and national certification criteria for midwives met with little notable response. Although there was no official vote that day because the meeting was considered "informational" for the Joint Commission on Health Care's (JCHC) Midwifery Subcommittee, which had been tasked with deciding whether to recommend licensure for direct-entry midwives (DEMs), the midwifery supporters in attendance left feeling weary and frustrated. To lighten our spirits, we retreated to a local pizza parlor for a "strategy session" to organize for the next hearing, which was a few weeks away.

My ethnographic fieldwork with midwifery supporters in Virginia began just after midwifery organizers had convinced legislators to institute a study of midwives by the JCHC in 1998 and continued through the passage of legislation to license certified professional midwives (CPMs) in 2005. The successful grassroots organizing of midwives and their supporters became immediately apparent in the overwhelming support for midwives documented by the JCHC Midwifery Subcommittee. Of the sixty-three individuals who spoke at public meetings throughout the state, sixty-one spoke in favor of legalizing DEMs. These included parents whose children's births had been attended by midwives, Virginia's only legally practicing DEM at the time (who had been "grandmothered" in when laws changed in the 1970s), several CNMs, and representatives of grassroots organizations supporting midwifery.[9] Despite a medical lobbyist's plea for physician participation in this process "to get reasonable legislation . . . on direct-entry midwives" in a publication by the Virginia Obstetrical and Gynecological Society (VA OB/GYN Society) and the Virginia Chapter of the American College of Obstetricians and Gynecologists (VA-ACOG),[10] only two representatives from these groups spoke at public hearings, and only one representative from the Medical Society of Virginia (MSV) sent a letter opposing legislation.[11] In total, the JCHC received comments from 192 people, 183 of which explicitly supported the licensure of CPMs.[12] Further, "Following the public comments period, the Joint Commission also received a petition signed by 124 citizens requesting 'the General Assembly to decriminalize the practice of home-based midwifery. This includes legalizing the Certified Professional Midwife.'"[13]

The JCHC ultimately recommended legislation that would legalize the practice of direct-entry midwifery by individuals who met the requirements of the North American Registry of Midwives (NARM) for certification as CPMs.[14] NARM is the primary national certifying body for DEMs,[15] and NARM's CPM certification allows for "multiple educational routes of entry, including apprenticeship, self-study, private midwifery schools, college- and university-based midwifery programs and nurse-midwifery."[16] As Davis-Floyd has explained, "Where you gained your knowledge, skills, and experience is not the issue—that you have them is what counts."[17] Nevertheless, to become a CPM, an applicant must "complete a clinical component that is at least one year in length and equivalent to 1,350 contact hours under the supervision of one or more approved preceptors" and must pass a written and clinical examination.[18] Additionally, recertification is required every three years.

Midwifery organizers in Virginia drafted several bills, which were introduced during the three years following the JCHC's midwifery study. Each of these subsequent bills, facing strong opposition from VA-ACOG,[19] the MSV, the Virginia Department of Health, the Department of Health Professions, and the state's chief medical examiner, was rejected in committee before reaching the floor of the full House or Senate. While the JCHC had recommended that a bill be introduced to legalize the CPM, the fact that they gave no seal of approval to any particular piece of legislation became a disadvantage to midwifery supporters.[20]

It was during this time period (2000–2002) that homebirth mothers stood at the forefront of public advocacy for DEMs. As a result of the intensified investigations of midwives, documented in Chapter 3, Virginia midwives remained relatively quiet on the political front during early efforts to legalize their practice. After the statute that prohibited DEMs was struck down in

2003, however, midwives became more public in their legislative efforts, as I discuss further at the conclusion of this chapter. Here, however, I focus on a three-year-period, during which bills to license CPMs failed in the Virginia legislature, and I examine in detail the struggles that *homebirth mothers* faced in the legislative arena.

Vilifying Mothers

Medical and state officials have historically justified state regulation and the medical management of reproductive healthcare by highlighting the "pathological" practices of mothers, particularly mothers who challenge dominant American trends and ideologies of childbirth.[21] By accusing mothers of "bad" behavior toward their children, medical officials have frequently been able to convince legislators that they are better equipped to make decisions regarding childbirth and mothering practices than the mothers they deem delinquent. In this way, medical officials have assigned pregnancy, birth, and motherhood to the "public" domain, and thus subjected mothers to surveillance (and discipline) by both medical institutions and the state.[22] What constituted "good" childbirth decisions and respectable mothering practices, however, were not always clear. For example, conflicting advice from medical experts about breastfeeding versus formula feeding has often put mothers in a precarious position; whether they choose to breastfeed or use heavily marketed infant formula, they are often chastised for not doing what is "right" for their children.[23] The construction of what is and what is not considered respectable mothering was also fiercely disputed in the Virginia legislature as public debate ensued over midwifery.

For a three year-period, 2000–2002, attending members of the Health, Welfare, and Institutions (HWI) Committee listened to fifteen minutes of testimony from both opponents and proponents of bills to license DEMs before defeating these bills. Opponents included representatives of the VA OB/GYN Society, the VA-ACOG, and the MSV. Proponents included representatives of grassroots organizations supporting midwifery, CPMs who had practiced legally in other states, and supportive CNMs. After each presentation, delegates were given time to ask speakers questions regarding the specifics of their presentation and the bill more generally. On several occasions, these questions provoked lengthy conversations about the safety and risks of homebirth, the training of midwives and, as I highlight in this chapter, the rights of parents (particularly mothers) to choose appropriate healthcare for their children.

It would be an oversimplification of the legislative process—as well as the persuasiveness of unregulated campaign contributions by well-funded medical organizations and individual physicians in Virginia[24]—to consider any of these examples the single "defining argument" that won the case for opponents of midwifery legislation during these years. However, it was clear that legislators gave at least tacit approval through nods and affirmative gestures when medical officials presented "commonsense" arguments that linked the medical management of childbirth to governmental control over mothering practices. In contrast, as evidenced in my first experience in the legislature, politicians were generally inattentive to the presentations of midwifery supporters. During the 2000 HWI Committee hearing, for instance, proponents of the legislation to license CPMs elected to speak first. At the beginning of the midwifery supporters' testimony, only four of the twenty-two delegates were in the hearing room. Fourteen others trickled in as the presentations proceeded, but less than half heard any testimony supporting the bill to license CPMs. In subsequent years, midwifery supporters opted to give their testimony after the opposition to ensure that delegates were at least present to hear it.

"Birth Is, by Nature, a Medical Event": Medical Authority as "Common Sense"

In the first HWI Committee hearing regarding CPM licensure in 2000, Dr. John Partridge, a representative of the VA OB/GYN Society and VA-ACOG, spoke in opposition to the bill. He began his presentation by touting the medical advances in maternity care over the past hundred years:

> Modern medicine has brought maternity care to an ever-safer level and loosening the standard would place mothers and babies at risk. . . . Birth is, by nature, a medical event. /In contrast, homebirth is/ a slippery slope, like driving a car without brakes. You may do okay on level ground with no turns, but when the road starts going downhill, and you start making some turns, it gets very dicey. . . . Isn't it logical to think hospitals and doctors have made birth safer? /I hope that you will/ preserve the public health of mothers and babies by preserving the current statutes. You'll hear mothers talk about preserving their right to choose, but I ask you, what about the baby's choice?[25]

Drawing on his confidence in medical superiority over childbirth, Partridge primed his audience for his "commonsense" assertion: *Birth is, by nature, a medical event.* Thus when Partridge invoked *nature* as an analogy for medicalized childbirth (meaning physician-attended hospital births, which have only occurred for just over a century), he spoke of assumed societal standards of risk in childbirth. His analogy, which linked *driving a car without brakes* to the dangers he associated with homebirth, served as additional reinforcement of the authority and hierarchy of the medical system by applying to midwife homebirths the long-established medical metaphor of the body as machine and the physician as mechanic.[26] Clearly, Partridge suggested, CPMs lacked the "tools" to deal with labor complications.

In her research on authoritative knowledge in obstetrics and midwifery, Brigitte Jordan has described how the ascendance and legitimation of the medical model as *the* authoritative knowledge system around healthcare and childbirth in much of the world have resulted in the devaluation of alternative knowledge systems as backward, naïve, and potentially troublesome. What is so persuasive about medicine as authoritative knowledge, then, is that "it seems natural, reasonable, and consensually constructed."[27] Therefore, it came as no surprise when Partridge stated, commonsensically, that homebirth mothers take unnecessary risks when they choose to give birth outside of the hospital: *Isn't it logical to think that hospitals and doctors have made birth safer?*[28] In answer to his rhetorical question, Partridge asked lawmakers to join him to *preserve the public health of mothers and babies*, linking his role as a physician and the state's role as protector of the health of its citizens. Thus Partridge's claim implicitly reinforces the benevolence of a government that regulates women's bodies by allowing medical dominance over reproduction.[29] Yet his phrasing of his position as a question to legislators (and, presumably, the broader assembled audience) allows "all participants [to] come to see the current social order [as] the way things (obviously) are."[30] Partridge's strategy was doubly effective because the statement placed the power and authority of good outcomes with both physicians and legislators, while bad outcomes remained the responsibility of the mother (as we saw against African American mothers historically in Chapter 3 and we will see again and again in more recent legislative debates).

Partridge also countered women's right to choose homebirth with a familiar slogan from the pro-life movement: *What about the baby's choice?* This final statement drew attention to connections between efforts to gain access to midwives and other reproductive rights activism, in this case "fetal rights" efforts in the pro-life movement. Political scientist Rachel Roth has written extensively on how fetal rights arguments have ultimately been used to restrict women's rights in childbirth, including forcing women to undergo unwanted medical procedures, such as court-ordered cesarean sections, for what legal and medical officials believe to be in the best interests of the women's *babies*, as Partridge argued earlier.[31] Although pro-life midwifery proponents would likely stop short of applying this argument to a woman's desire to homebirth, invoking "fetal rights" has been an effective strategy for midwifery opponents.

It is also important to remember that midwifery supporters are deeply divided over a woman's "right to choose" an abortion and, as sociologists Wendy Simonds, Barbara Katz Rothman, and Bari Meltzer Norman have explained,

"For midwives [and their supporters] who oppose abortion, dedication to 'choice' does not extend to all procreative issues. Once a pregnancy occurs, they support procreative decision making about who, when, where, and how prenatal care and birth will occur—but not whether or not to continue the pregnancy."[32] As Pamela Klassen has discussed more broadly in her writing about the complicated relationship between religion, homebirth, and women's reproductive rights activism:

> Arguments against homebirth that belittle women's experiences of birth (of the "if you want an experience, ride a roller coaster" variant) and refuse to acknowledge women's right and responsibility to choose their desired place to give birth, fit along a continuum with . . . fetal rights arguments. They downplay a woman's role and experience giving birth in place of emphasizing the "outcome" of the baby. However, in a society that proclaims passionate interest in healthy babies, but then fails to find solutions to the problems of child poverty once those babies age, these are not so much positive arguments guarding the baby as they are negative arguments circumscribing the autonomy of the birthing woman.[33]

Partridge's invocation of "logic," "nature," and the "common sense" of medical authority over childbirth remained central to medical officials' attacks against homebirth—and, more importantly, homebirth mothers—in subsequent years.

"In Homebirths Either Myself or My Children Would Have Been at Risk": Medically Managed Childbirth as a Claim to Respectable American Motherhood

Dr. Anne Peterson, commissioner of the Virginia Department of Health, coordinated the testimony of the opposition to the bill that was reintroduced to legalize the licensure of CPMs in the 2001 HWI Committee hearing. She opened the opposition's commentary by emphasizing her own position as a mother who made the mainstream choice to deliver her children in the hospital. An important feature in the personal testimony and childbirth stories offered by female physicians was that they were able to speak authoritatively about childbirth and motherhood as both physicians *and* respectable mothers.[34] Female medical officials relied on their own experience of childbirth and motherhood to question the legitimacy of homebirth mothers' childbirth decisions. In the following excerpt, Peterson used her own experience in childbirth to reaffirm Partridge's statement from the previous year, that homebirth mothers' decisions can endanger their own and their babies' lives. Further, Peterson places homebirth mothers outside of the cadre of normal *American* mothers who accept the medical management of labor and delivery as the only way to reduce the risks associated with childbirth.

> I myself had low-risk pregnancies and high-risk deliveries and in home births either myself or my children would have been at risk. . . . /Birth/ is a place where Americans have spoken very strongly about their willingness to take on risk relative to deliveries. OB/GYN doctors pay more malpractice [insurance] than most other physicians, and family practitioners who do labor and delivery services pay more than family practitioners who do not do it. So, Americans have really spoken to the amount of risk they are willing to accept in this arena.[35]

Peterson separated homebirth mothers from *American* mothers who acknowledged high risks in pregnancy by their willingness to go to the hospital (and to file lawsuits when things went awry, as indicated by rising malpractice rates). She also implied that homebirth mothers did not accurately assess the risks associated with childbirth and did not uphold *American* values when they refused to follow mainstream childbirth trends to lessen those dangers.[36]

The strategy of rebuking homebirth mothers for their inability to assess risk was also common among physicians who were seeking to eliminate midwives in the early 1900s. For example, early twentieth-century medical reports in Virginia berated African American women for their "inattention" to their prenatal care, their "failure" to report "danger signals" during pregnancy, and their "insensibility" to the health of their newborns.[37] The mothers' "failure" or "insensibility" was often considered a result of their continued use of midwives, particularly among poor women, as segregated hospital clinics became available to middle-class and affluent African Americans in the mid-1900s. Few of these reports addressed the economic impoverishment and lack of access to basic healthcare services in African American communities, which remain key factors in high infant and maternal mortality statistics.[38] In contrast, medical reports at the turn of the twenty-first century also rarely mention the relatively good health of most contemporary homebirth mothers, or the better-than-average health of their babies.[39]

"It Only Takes One Bad Baby": Constructing the Choice to Homebirth as Pathological Motherhood

Throughout the debate over legalizing DEMs in Virginia, physicians maintained that mothers who elected to homebirth were bad mothers. For example, the president of the VA-OB/GYN Society, Dr. Willette LeHew, explained to lawmakers in 2000, "I call homebirth the earliest form of child abuse."[40] As the public debates raged on from 2000 to 2002, the medical opposition became more insistent that state and medical officials were more competent than mothers and parents to judge the "best interests" of Virginia's children.

In the 2002 HWI Committee hearing regarding several bills to license DEMs through different state regulatory structures,[41] a state delegate asked Dr. Steven Bentheim, a representative of VA-ACOG and the VA-OB/GYN Society, "But doctor, any patient has the right to consent to treatment, and if it is a minor child, then I, as the parent, am the one responsible for giving consent for that minor unless you want to go through a legal process to take my parental rights away. That is the current law, am I correct?" In response, Bentheim considered the mother's choice to homebirth (not just the practice of midwifery, which was common in other states) a pathological behavior by linking it to criminal acts, such as negligent motherhood and illegal drug use.

> I think that sometimes uh- that the mother's decision to deliver at home is not always in the baby's best interest, although, I think she might think it is. I'm not sure it is. . . . I do think that we also have to have minimal requirements over parents in the care of their children. We don't let them be-, in the news, a parent that goes to the store and leaves her child at home, the house burns down, she, you know, it was her prerogative to leave the child at home while she went. She thought that it was okay for the child to do so, but she is then-, you know Social Services or whoever may come in and investigate that. She may be /responsible/ or something. So, I think, once again, we have to-, hopefully try to find what we think is in the best interest of the mother and also in the best interests of the child. . . . But life is precious. And I'm telling you that these are children and it only takes one bad baby, or two bad babies to make you realize-. . . . I'm trying to think of how to say this uh, I'm not sure that just because it is going to happen that you have to-, you have to go along with it. Just the same way that we don't legalize drugs and I mean we don't say "okay, you know what, people are going to use drugs" and again this is probably a bad analogy

again, but people are going to make decisions for themselves and they're going to do it even though it isn't in their best interest.[42]

In his answer to the delegate's question about the rights of *parents* regarding their children's healthcare, it is notable that Bentheim, in his response, shifted to the use of a feminine pronoun. He invoked the idea of the pathological *parent that goes to the store* who leaves *her* child unattended, therefore specifying the mother as the negligent or bad parent. The mother's departure from the private space of the home is also important when she *leaves her child at home to go to the store*. Ultimately, a public state body, S*ocial Services or whatever,* must intervene in the mother's private space to investigate whether she may be held *responsible* and to ensure her good, state-sanctioned mothering behavior. This reprimand effectively argued against women's legal right to make mothering and childbirth choices in the home by linking homebirth mothers to negligent mothers.

Additionally, Bentheim's critical assessment of the unidentified *them* in the beginning of his answer extended his opposition to midwifery by calling on both physicians and the state to protect Virginians: *We have to do what is in the best interests of the mother and the child.* Bentheim emphasized the role of legislators *and* physicians in regulating the mothering practices and, by extension, the birthing practices of potentially negligent mothers. He also transitioned from talking about *a/the mother* neglecting *her/the children* in the last passage to the potential hazards that mothers pose to their *babies,* drawing on the sympathy of the audience regarding a mother who would choose an alternative (deemed unsafe for her baby) to a mainstream childbirth practice. In fact, he cautioned against producing *bad babies* instead of, perhaps, bad outcomes, which further conveyed the pathology he attributed to homebirth mothers onto their children. As Susan Hyatt suggests in her study of the medicalization of motherhood among impoverished women in Britain, medical and state officials often identify the mother "not primarily as an individual in her own right but . . . the conduit through which her children [are] to be made into productive and healthy citizens of the state (or not)."[43] Therefore, if a mother is considered risky or otherwise deemed unfit, then this could potentially be passed along to her children. Similarly, Virginia state representatives commonly referred not only to "illegal births" by homebirth mothers (which is inaccurate, because women are legally entitled to birth wherever they choose in the United States) but also to "illegal babies," presumably those babies born into the hands of midwives.[44] Thus officials suggested that because homebirth mothers engaged in what they (erroneously) believed to be an illegal act, the mothers' criminality would then be passed on to their children.

Along a similar line of reasoning, Bentheim's equation of *people* who *are going to use drugs* and *people* who are going to *make decisions for themselves*, presumably to homebirth, shows how he linked negligent mothers, illegal drug users, and homebirth mothers. Ultimately, Bentheim implied a connection between individual women's "bad choices" regarding childbirth and the health of society at large by likening homebirth to practices that most audience members (including state delegates and homebirth proponents) would consider bad choices. This strategy effectively allowed Bentheim to mark homebirth as a symptom of pathological motherhood and, simultaneously, a practice to be restricted by legislators.

Of course, the view that women who do not follow mainstream childbirth norms are "bad" mothers and "bad" citizens,[45] and that the state and medical powers work hand in hand to scrutinize and discipline them, is not new. One revealing example is the experience of drug-addicted mothers in Florida, where the state mandates jail sentences for women who are tested and found positive for certain drugs during their pregnancies. Ironically, once they are incarcerated, the state punishes these women (and their fetuses) further by denying them both prenatal care and addiction treatment while they serve out their jail terms. Thus some drug-addicted women attempt to protect themselves from going to jail by avoiding prenatal care. They are then identified by the state as criminally negligent mothers and can be charged with child abuse.[46] This example epitomizes the way medical institutions, such as hospitals and clinics, and government institutions, such as public health agencies and the court system, collude to discipline women who do not fit the model of "good American mothers."[47] Although I would hardly equate homebirth with drug addiction during pregnancy, as Bentheim seemed content to do in front of the Virginia General Assembly, both examples illuminate how derogatory stereotypes about mothers who attempt to protect themselves and their children outside of state-sanctioned models are used to devalue their status as good mothers and citizens.

Reclaiming Respectable Motherhood

Midwifery supporters' testimony during the 2000–2002 legislative hearings marked a significant departure from medical definitions of respectable motherhood. Speakers in favor of the legislation presented studies on the safety of homebirth and outlined the CPM's extensive training while they simultaneously attempted to counter claims by medical officials that homebirthers were bad mothers. Midwifery supporters' frustration with the portrayal of homebirthing women as pathological mothers and the disregard of their rights to make legal choices about where and with whom they gave birth were

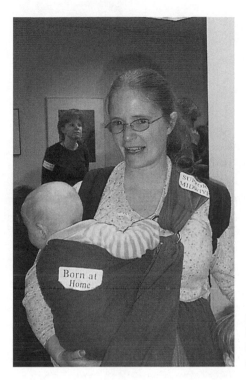

Figure 4.1   Homebirth mother, Sally Holdener, with her "Born at Home" baby in the legislature. *(Photo by the author, 2005)*

dominant themes in their testimony. Joining the formal presenters were other homebirth mothers—frequently between twenty and sixty women—who had traveled, often with multiple children in tow, from areas throughout the state to support midwifery legislation. They made their support known by wearing buttons to support midwives and by putting stickers on their children that boasted "Born at Home" or "Born into the Loving Hands of a Midwife," symbols of the sensible choices they had made in electing to have a midwife-attended homebirth (see figure 4.1).

"We've Decided for Ourselves and Our Babies": Mothers as Educated Consumers

Speaking for the grassroots pro-midwifery organization Virginia Birthing Freedom in an HWI Committee meeting, Ellen Hamblet formally challenged opponents' claims against homebirth and homebirth mothers. Hamblet, similar to the female doctors who relied on their own status as mothers, as well as their professional credentials, to bolster their claims, presented herself as a mother concerned with the safety of her children, alongside her professional credentials—her service in the U.S. Navy and her position as the co-director of a grassroots pro-midwifery organization. Challenging physicians' assumptions of what "normal" Americans desire in childbirth, Hamblet argued that women who desire homebirth are indeed *concerned with the health and safety of babies* and, by extension, they are also normal, respectable American citizens.

> When it comes down to the bottom line, we are all, everybody in this room, concerned with the health and safety of babies. So, we should be able to start with this bottom line and build something that we all can be proud of as a way, as Dr. Peterson said, to support midwives in Virginia, and also to allow families to make the informed legal choice to have their babies at home, to be able to hire a midwife. . . . Most of us never have the occasion to even wonder about whether the hospital is a safe place to be in birth. That's the way we do it in this country. That's the way most of us did it for our first pregnancies. Most women never have a chance to come back and question that decision, never have reason to come back and question it because their experience in the hospital is great. They have a great doctor, they have a great hospital, everything works the way it's supposed to be, they feel well served by the system. Those are not the women in this room today. We are mostly women who have gone and have had bad experiences with hospital birth and feel that these experiences were unnecessarily dangerous, that they were at a minimum disrespectful, and they scared us and made us feel that this is not the place we wanted to go necessarily for birth. . . . I'll tell you, we're a bunch of moms here and what we know is that we've done a lot of research, that we've decided for ourselves and our babies that we want to have a homebirth. We're telling you that we need to be able to hire a midwife to do that. We're telling you that we can't hire midwives right now because there is no path, there's no way to do that in Virginia . . . legally. And so, we're telling you that we need your help.[48]

Unlike physicians' accounts of risky and ill-informed mothers, Hamblet portrayed homebirth parents as normal American *moms* who had rationally chosen to question childbirth in the hospital, especially after their negative experiences during previous births. Hamblet challenged the commonsense logic that all births are *medical events* that need to be attended by physicians in hospitals. Instead, she explained that homebirth mothers have *done a lot of research* and *want to be able to hire a midwife*. The year before she had explained to legislators in more explicit terms that mothers, as "consumers" of midwifery services, were "caught in the middle of poor relations between doctors and midwives" when they could not access the practitioners they desired.[49]

Focusing on the logic and rationality of homebirth mothers' concerns, Hamblet concluded by asking for the state's protection regarding women's legal right to choose homebirth. By countering medical challenges that suggested homebirth mothers' negligence or insensibility regarding the welfare of their children, Hamblet attempted to legitimate not only homebirth but also the responsible decision-making strategies of homebirth mothers. She characterized homebirthers as respectable American mothers, precisely because of their pragmatic decisions regarding childbirth and the health of their children, especially after experiencing *dangerous* and *disrespectful* treatment in the hospital. Just like all respectable American mothers, she argued, homebirth mothers want what they consider the safest choice for themselves *and* their babies.

Speaking again the following year, Hamblet personalized her defense of homebirth as a respectable childbirth choice for Virginia mothers by vindicating her own good mothering practices as a homebirth mother.

> We believe that birth is healthy, birth is sacred, and hospitals do not do it justice and are best avoided unless they're needed for complications. But then, I'm just a mom, so what do I know? I'm the person who is responsible for this baby's health and future every minute of every day, with every choice I make. But can I also be trusted to know the best place for this baby to be born, and to decide who is the best care provider for us?[50]

Hamblet's sarcastic rhetorical question indicates the frustration that she also communicated in a Listserv post after prior defeats:

> The Va Medical Society and the Va Chapter of Obstetricians and Gynecologists played on emotion (since realistically there's not much logic they can use against midwives and home birth). They scared the legislators into thinking that legalizing midwives would in some way endanger babies (let's not even consider what went down behind the scenes talking about $$$). That's a trump card . . . if legislators feel (or can say they feel) that they're protecting babies from the bad decisions made by their selfish mothers (grrrr), all the logic in the world won't prevail against that.[51]

Attesting to her broader status as a normal American mother, Hamblet includes herself among the group of other "good American mothers" who care for and desire the best for their babies when using the term *this baby* instead of *my baby* in front of legislative delegates. By extension, she argues that her political actions to gain access to homebirth do not, in fact, negate her mothering skills and commitment to her children but instead support her desires for the *best care provider for us.*

Hamblet was not alone in her dissatisfaction with medical officials' portrayal of homebirth mothers in the legislature. Although other midwifery supporters did not respond formally within the General Assembly, many wrote letters to delegates, newspaper editors, and even the opposing physicians. Midwifery supporters also responded privately to the charges leveled against them, both on Listservs and in conversations with each other, which I discuss further in Chapter 5.

Continuing the Struggle: Legislative Successes, 2003–2005

In 2003, midwifery organizers were successful in their efforts to strike down the 1976 statute that had made it illegal for everyone except CNMs—and the few non-nurse midwives who had been "grandmothered" in—to provide midwifery services. Notably, the decision was made rather quietly, with little opposition from medical officials and without the heated public debates that characterized legislative hearings regarding previous midwifery bills. The reasons for this change were open to speculation among midwifery supporters, but state and medical officials later made it clear that rescinding the 1976 law did not protect midwives against charges of "practicing medicine without a license" or "practicing nurse-midwifery without a license." Prior to the passage of legislation to license CPMs in 2005, midwives and their supporters expressed continued concerns over the legal safety of DEMs, especially as medical officials continued to fight diligently against subsequent bills to license CPMs and legislators rejected bills aimed at licensure in 2003 and 2004.

After the legislative change in 2003, however, DEMs became more politically visible and became the primary speakers advocating for their professional licensure at legislative hearings. A bill to license CPMs made it through Virginia's House of Representatives in 2004, but it was rejected by the Senate Committee on Education and Health after a physician asserted, familiarly, that licensing midwives "would not be in the best interests of the women and children of Virginia."[52] Notably, Senator Janet Howell waited until just before this vote to tell an unsettling personal story.[53] Although she had decided on a hospital delivery in 1969, she explained that her friend, who was seeing the same obstetrician, had desired a home delivery.[54] When the women went into labor at the same time, they both had to go to the hospital to ensure that the obstetrician could be in attendance for both deliveries. The senator's friend had complications but was treated successfully in the hospital. Afterward, the physician credited the coincidence of the senator's labor, which required the other woman to come to the hospital, with saving the homebirth-bound woman's life. The senator closed the story by relaying the physician's decision never to attend another homebirth. By the senator's account, her prudent childbirth choices saved the life of her unknowing friend, as well as any other homebirther mothers who might have followed in her footsteps with this physician. She characterized her vote against the bill to license CPMs as an extension of her efforts to protect Virginia mothers from making "bad" choices. It is clear that despite the increased participation of midwives in the legislative debates over their practice in Virginia, anecdotes implying that mothers who chose homebirth were uninformed, or reckless, remained convincing arguments in efforts to restrict the practice of midwives.

Despite these continued setbacks, legislation to license CPMs was successful in 2005 (see figure 4.2). Importantly, the bill ensured independent practice for CPMs and did not require mothers to be assessed by another healthcare professional in order to seek midwifery care. Thus the "physician supervision"

Figure 4.2 Two newly licensed CPMs from Virginia, Leslie Payne and Cathi Barrett, at a Midwives Alliance of North America Conference. *(Photo by the author, 2006)*

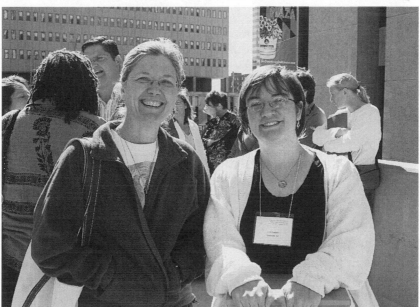

requirement, which prevents out-of-hospital practice for many nurse-midwives in Virginia, does not affect CPMs under this law.[55] One drawback of this bill, however, was that it prohibited the possession and administration of controlled substances, including oxygen, which national groups, such as NARM, recommend in homebirth settings. Most midwives and their supporters argued, however, that this was acceptable in order to pass the CPM licensure bill, and that these and other regulations would be reconsidered in future years (see the Epilogue for further discussion).

Thus midwives and their supporters were ecstatic about the law and saw the passage of this legislation as evidence that their hard work lobbying legislators over an eight-year period had been worthwhile. Still, the dissatisfaction and disempowerment that many midwifery supporters have felt from both medical and state authorities highlight their understanding of a state and medical community in coalition that opposes a group of vulnerable women vying for their reproductive rights. In this context of hostility I found that most homebirth mothers identify themselves as not being "politically active," despite their diligent work to support midwives in their communities and throughout the state.

In part, this avoidance of a politicized identity may have to do with the long-term tensions between midwifery advocates and the self-consciously political activists within the reproductive rights movement. However, the language that midwifery supporters use in legislative debates, in organizing efforts, and in my interviews with them regarding their support for midwives suggests that the emerging identity of "midwifery consumer" also plays a role. In their effort to present themselves as respectable American mothers—countering decades of medical and legislative hostility toward homebirthers—consumer identity offered a politically palatable option for many midwifery supporters, but at the same time it inhibited a more politicized identity as activists working for changes in reproductive healthcare. By definition, a consumer interacts with the state through the act of consuming various goods and services, not in her or his capacity as a citizen activist working to *change* the existing system. Thus it was not surprising that many of the homebirthers I interviewed told me that they were not explicitly political . . . but that they were often heavily involved in efforts to support midwives—both legislatively and in their local communities.

5

"I'm Not Really Politically Active, but..."

Negotiating Political Identity and "Activist Mothering"

Activist mothering . . . involves nurturing work for those
outside one's kinship group, but [it] also encompasses a
broad definition of actual mothering practices. . . . [In this
sense,] "good mothering" [can] comprise all actions,
including social activism, that address . . . the needs of
[women's] children and community.
—NANCY NAPLES, GRASSROOTS WARRIORS

In light of medical and legislative efforts to discredit homebirth mothers, it comes as little surprise that many midwifery supporters in my study hesitated to identify themselves as overtly politically active in their struggle for midwives. Apprehension over the state's response to an explicitly political identity was of particular concern for women from low-income backgrounds who shared fears of losing their children if government officials were to disapprove of their parenting or birthing choices. Many middle-class midwifery supporters responded differently to the damaging stereotypes, however, by arguing that they were indeed respectable mothers, precisely *because* they were active in the political process, pursuing what they believed was best for them and their children. Although many of these women, like lower-income women, declared that they were *not* "politically active," and few would have described themselves as "activist mothers," they were likely to cite trips to the legislature as ultimately "empowering" and "energizing" experiences. Accordingly, middle-class and affluent women also began to redefine themselves as consumers (rather than as citizens or activists) to highlight *their* economic power in the face of the well-paid lobbyists, physicians, and public health officials who represented the medical societies and the government. Low-income women, however, did not find consumer identification comforting, as they continued to struggle with the fear of state intervention in their lives for making "bad" consumer choices (such as having a homebirth) and the vulnerability many experienced in medical settings (in addition to the disrespect that all homebirth mothers were subject to in the legislature). Despite these fears, however, low-income women were frequently engaged in "everyday" forms of activism—similar to the efforts of the "activist mothers" that Nancy Naples describes in *Grassroots Warriors*—that contributed to their struggle for access to midwives in their communities.

Women's Political Identities: Redefining "Politics"

Similar to homebirth mothers' efforts to portray themselves as apolitical mothers in the face of medical and state criticism, feminist scholars have shown that women in a variety of social movements and community struggles have redefined their political experiences as an extension of their family roles as wives, mothers, and daughters, rather than as an activist work.[1] Yet as anthropologist Sandra Morgen has written in her research on working-class women's activism for women's healthcare:

> Women's community-based political activism is a conscious and collective way of expressing and acting on their interests as *women*, as *wives and mothers*, as *members of neighborhoods and communities*, and as *members of particular race, ethnic, and class groups*. To collapse a complex political consciousness into the more narrow confines of domestic values, interests and roles is to distort both the motivation and the political implications of this mode of resistance.[2]

Naples, a sociologist, has called this strategy "activist mothering," through which women extend their nurturing of their families toward their communities, drawing on "traditional female identities to justify taking revolutionary action to improve their community and the lives of their family."[3] This "community caretaking," Naples argues, is often overlooked by scholars of politics and political activism because it falls outside of legislative and electoral politics.

Feminists have argued for several decades that politics and political activism need to be redefined to understand women's participation in social change efforts.[4] In short, they suggest that we depart from analyses that focus solely on electoral and legislative arenas, where men's influence has long predominated, to include what women do in their local communities. Echoing Naples's description of "activist mothering," the stories that homebirth mothers told me about their support of midwives "counter traditional constructions of politics as limited to electoral politics or membership in social movement organizations."[5]

Women's strategy of claiming to avoid "politics" is also not a new one.[6] In fact, women active in political struggles have frequently avoided defining themselves as political activists, even when this denial is in direct contrast to their actions toward social change. For example, many women reject the label "feminist" but develop ideas and participate in actions that "fall within the repertoire of feminism."[7] Similarly, the community-based political activities of the women Naples described as "activist mothers" often did not fit within their own conception of "politics."

> Most . . . did not define themselves as political people, feminists, rad-icals, or socialists . . . they simply believed they were acting to protect their communities.
>
> Simultaneously, they held a radical critique of establishment politics that contested the dominant definitions of "the political" and accurately saw the limitations of dialogue with and incorporations into the dominant political system. Because the [women] believed that politics was a formal system by which wealthy men (and, sometimes, women) vied for power for its own sake, they distinguished themselves from politicians who they viewed as out for their own gain.[8]

Similarly, the relationships that women in my study described between homebirth mothers and state and medical officials ultimately soured their willingness (and sometimes ability) to engage in legislative battles.

The socioeconomic differences among homebirthers were also relevant to the way in which women presented their relationships to the state. Even before I spoke to those who agreed to participate in my study, or asked them about their educational levels or income, their various levels of access to resources were apparent. Most participants had generously invited me into their homes to conduct interviews. In one instance, I drove up to a Federal-style mansion, complete with manicured gardens, for a quick interview before the midwifery supporter had to leave for a series of afternoon appointments. Another participant lived with her husband and five children in a modest three-bedroom house, with rooms in various stages of renovation and sheets hung as partitions to offer privacy. One woman lived with her newborn in a newly renovated townhouse at the center of a bustling small town and made it a point to explain that the confederate flag that hung over the Ikea furniture in her living room reminded her of "her roots."

Another homebirther gave me a tour of her spacious new home in a suburban development. She was particularly fond of her three children's "themed" bedrooms, each professionally decorated with fire engines, clowns, and ballerinas. Two other homebirthers lived in homes that they were proud to have built themselves—with the help of friends and family in their community—from salvaged wood and unpainted siding. One of these families had an extensive organic garden and lived in an open-air home without electricity or running water. The other family was proud to share their new solar-powered shower with me when they invited me to stay with them, and to point out the "beautiful mama wren" who flew in and out of the unscreened windows to bring her new babies grubs atop their living room bookshelf. Although most of the women I interviewed and stayed with in each of these locations described themselves as vulnerable in regard to state and medical officials, their levels of vulnerability—and the ways in which they expressed their concerns—were frequently quite different.

"It Is a Gathering of Women in the Face of Men in Suits": Vulnerable Mothers

Nearly all of the participants in my study expressed a sense of disempowerment as homebirth mothers by both the state and the healthcare system. Indeed, their choice to homebirth had been contested publicly in the Virginia legislature. Many midwifery supporters explained that their role as mothers, and certainly as homebirthers, seemed out of place in this domain. Many felt that legislators and medical officials thought of them as too *insignificant*,[9] too *fringe*,[10] too *extreme, radical*,[11] *too ignorant, stupid, naïve*,[12] and *not sophisticated* enough[13] to demand rights through political actions. One homebirth mother, Theresa Neal, shared her experience in the legislature after she had traveled several hours from her rural community to attend a legislative hearing with her midwife.

It was a thrill to be in Richmond, playing with the big guys, you know, the legislators, but they made me really angry most of the time because they were clueless and they didn't come to meetings and they hadn't read anything and they were voting on my life and they were not informed and that really upset me. . . . It's always been about power. And right now it's about power because the people in the medical community and who support the medical community are completely— choose to be completely ignorant of the facts. . . . And it is very much a gender thing for me because if you look at the people going to Rich-

mond, there are certainly plenty of dads there and dads are taking care
of kids so the moms can go there and that kind of thing, but it is a
gathering of women. It is a gathering of women in the face of men in
suits in the legislature and I find it to be so stark in contrast. And these
men telling us what is safe and what is not safe when they have not
been through it is so offensive.[14]

Theresa linked her frustration with legislators and physicians to her broader
understanding of the gendered oppression that women face in both the medical and legislative arena. She also drew attention to the importance of wom-
en's personal experience and the knowledge gained through the experience of
childbirth, in contrast to *the big guys, legislators* and *people in the medical community.* Taken together, she described these *men in suits* as *not informed, ignorant, clueless,* and *offensive* (which she reiterates). During our interview, Theresa similarly criticized female legislators and physicians who were equally as
inattentive (and often rude) to homebirth mothers. She emphasized the important power differences between women—particularly as they are disempowered as mothers and homebirthers—and both state and medical officials.

Other midwifery supporters likened their experience in the legislature to
being treated like children—not unlike the experiences many had had delivering their children in a hospital.[15] For example, Cindy Newton offered the
analogy of a parent-child relationship to describe state legislators' responses
to homebirth mothers.

They keep, you know, if the government means our legislature, they
keep saying "no," flat no, like a child saying, "I want a later curfew" or
something and the parent saying, "No, you can't have what you want.
You are not mature enough." . . . I mean, it's so insulting if you let yourself think what their approval really means. You know, it really means
they think we don't know any better. It really means that the government thinks that they know better than we do. And it's a paternalistic-,
even though some of them may be women, attitude of, "We know best
and you can't have this."[16]

Cindy suggested that *the government, our legislature,* and the metaphorical
parent are in opposition to the women and mothers they view as children. Like
many other midwifery supporters, she balked at the state's *paternalistic* and
parental role regarding mothers.

Another midwifery supporter, Paula Queen, used the potent metaphor of
being raped to describe both her experience of medicalized (hospital) childbirth and the *big hand of government* that was limiting her childbirth options:

I see it [my births in the hospital] very clearly as rape now. . . . It also makes me question myself that I was so blinded. . . . And I can't even mourn it. I could mourn it by myself, but there's not that many people that understand it. It's not like I can go report it to let you know you're standing up for yourself. . . . I see it as a crunch of the big hand of government coming down and doing that [forcing women to give birth in hospitals] and women not even knowing it . . . that they really are missing a part of them[selves].[17]

Most important to Paula was that women were not even recognizing that both the medical system and *the big hand of government* had taken away the power she felt women should gain through childbirth. In essence, Paula felt that women were being doubly raped by being forced to "choose" hospital birth, both by the political opposition of medical officials to midwifery legislation and by the government that had denied women the ability to legally choose a homebirth midwife. In this case, it is important to make a distinction between what anthropologist Iris Lopez has described as "a decision that is based on lack of alternatives versus one that is based on reproductive freedom. A decision is said to be more voluntary when it is based on a greater space of viable alternatives and the conditions that make this possible."[18] For Paula and many homebirth mothers, their "choices" in childbirth were significantly limited when the government did not allow them access to midwives.

Evie Diaz also expressed her frustration when she felt that citizens, in contrast to paid lobbyists, were discouraged from participating in the legislative process.

We would have to sit through so many other issues and we were the only citizens down there [in the Virginia General Assembly]. Everyone else-, were lobbyists who-, hired guns to go get something for their industry that was paying them to be there. And we were a buncha moms with an occasional dad. . . . And h-how insignificant we were viewed. I mean, it has been, well it's, it's, it's obstetrics all over. /We were/ so disrespected. They really did not want to see us and then somebody would pull a boob out or a baby would cry (laughing) or you know and they're just like "Oh, God?!" I mean, [Linda Darner] posted [to a Listserv] that you know "this is called confrontational po—, um lobbying" . . . and I'm like (smacks tongue on the roof of her mouth in a chiding manner), I'm thinking we've been pretty confrontational from the beginning just 'cause we showed up. They have not known what to do with us. We were told we had bad manners.[19]

Evie initially set up *we* to mean midwifery supporters or, more specifically, *citizens*. By downplaying the political importance of *citizens* as *a buncha moms with an occasional dad* against *lobbyists, everyone else,* and *hired guns* who are paid *to go get something for their industry that was paying them to be there,* Evie highlighted the importance of midwifery supporters as volunteers. Although the women (mainly) participated as volunteers, the (mainly) male legislators and lobbyists were paid to attend legislative hearings.[20]

Echoing the concerns of other midwifery supporters, that medical lobbyists and legislators viewed politically active mothers as *mothers with bad manners,* Evie used adjectives such as *insignificant, disrespected,* and *confrontational* to describe midwifery supporters in contrast to *hired,* paid medical lobbyists in the General Assembly. Activists often identify themselves in contrast to state officials. For example, Michael Brown, in his study of AIDS activists, noted, "In the citizens that we imagine, the voters, grassroots volunteers, and clients are recipients of [government] services, while the bureaucrats are paid employees, professionals, and experts inside of, and embodying, the state."[21] Although Evie first identified *they* as lobbyists, *they* quickly became an amalgamation of medical lobbyists and legislators when she suggested that *they really did not want to see us. And then somebody would pull a boob out or a baby would cry (laughing) or you know and they're just like 'Oh, God?!* Evie alluded to both medical lobbyists and state officials in this instance by suggesting their joint discomfort with an openly nursing mother and, more specifically, when she likened her experiences within the legislature to the disrespect that she and other women had experienced during hospital childbirth: *It's obstetrics all over. /We were/ SO disrespected.* Evie's equation of these groups is hardly surprising, as she and other midwifery supporters who were struggling for legislation to protect midwives had witnessed legislators who had sided, again and again, with the powerful medical lobby. In the context of these strained relationships, most homebirth mothers were reluctant to enter into legislative debates, and they were equally hesitant about identifying their non-legislative community support of midwives as a form of political activity.

"I'm Not Really Politically Active, but...": Shifting Definitions

Although all of the women in my study described participating in activities that they characterized as "political activity" in reference to others, nearly two-thirds claimed explicitly that they were *not* engaged in "political activity" themselves. Almost all of the women had participated in local grassroots organizations and coalitions that supported midwives: many had attended legislative and judicial hearings, about half had spoken or written letters to political representatives, several had given testimony at public hearings on midwifery, and a few had participated in public demonstrations. Some participants also described certain home-based activities as explicitly "political," such as talking to people in their community about having a homebirth, experiencing homebirth themselves, participating on local and national Listservs, signing petitions carried door-to-door or at local events, donating money to organizations that supported midwifery, reading and expanding their personal knowledge about homebirth, and attending a friend's homebirth. Although all participants had engaged in at least some of these activities in support of midwives, in their homes and communities as well as within state-level politics, most denied that their own actions were political.

For example, Nancy Davis, a young mother in a rural area of the state who had never been to the Virginia General Assembly in Richmond, explained:

> I just support [midwifery] in a very under-the-table sort of a spontaneous way. I sign papers that I see if there's ever petitions going around. I have called lobbyists or called congressmen [when] I get prompted, but I'm not very politically active.[22]

Although Nancy describes *not* being *very politically active*, despite her actions to support midwives within her local community, even midwifery supporters who had participated in legislative debates in Richmond denied ties to political activism. For example, Cindy, who had likened the legislator-homebirther relationship to one of an overbearing parent and child, and who was a longtime, well-known midwifery supporter who had spoken before lawmakers in Richmond on several occasions, revealed:

> I hate anything to do with politics and have to be carried kicking and screaming to testify before the Senate subcommittee hearing, but I get irritated enough to do it. And, I mean, for different people, different levels are comfortable. For me, no level is comfortable, I just wish I didn't have to deal with it, but I do and I will deal with it because I feel really strongly that you can't sit back and say, "Oh, why doesn't somebody do something?" I mean, you have to be one of the doers. But for myself, I really try and stay in the background. . . . I don't think of myself as a political activist, but I do call myself a birth advocate, a consumer advocate for women about childbirth.[23]

Cindy described herself as reluctant but still *irritated enough* to testify before the General Assembly, particularly to support women's right to homebirth.

Nevertheless, she continued to distinguish herself from what she later described as *other people* who did engage in *politics*, such as running for office or picketing for a cause. She was torn between being politically active outside of her home and community and honoring her personal wish to stay out of politics entirely. In this way, Cindy fluctuated between staying out of public politics (*I don't think of myself as a political activist*) and engaging in them because it was, as she later put it, "the right thing to do."

It is also interesting that Cindy preferred to describe herself as a *consumer advocate* to underscore her contention that reproductive health was a woman's choice, particularly since she was a grandmother who could no longer have children. The power she felt as an affluent "consumer" became increasingly evident when she confidently described her experiences in the legislature when she spoke to predominantly affluent male legislators. Recounting her testimony, Cindy declared, "'You must listen to us. We're your wives, we're your daughters, we're your sisters. We know what we're talking about. We know what we want and you must pay attention to us.'"[24] By drawing on the socioeconomic similarities she shared with many legislators and her position as a wealthy "consumer," Cindy felt certain that they would indeed *pay attention*. This was not the case for all midwifery supporters, however.

"What If Something Were to Happen?": Differing Experiences of Political Action

Despite the varied levels of participation in the political process that midwifery supporters reported—from signing petitions to support midwives in their communities to testifying before the state legislature—it is significant that most felt compelled to deny their association with "political activity." Clearly, *all* midwifery supporters were troubled by the hostile attacks they received within and outside of the legislature regarding not only their effort to support midwives but also their ability to effectively parent their children as they advocated for homebirth. Notably, of the few participants in my study who explicitly claimed to be politically active, all were either currently practicing midwives or were primary organizers in grassroots groups supporting midwifery. Most mothers who had experienced midwife-assisted homebirths downplayed the "political" nature of their contributions. Although at first I viewed the denial of political activity as a general trend among women who were disempowered in their efforts to support midwives, as I began to compare the responses of participants from different socioeconomic backgrounds, a more complicated pattern emerged. Although almost all of the women claimed they avoided political action, it became evident that they did so for very different reasons.

Sociologist Celene Krauss has noted differences between the ways in which white women and women of color who became involved in community struggles for environmental justice responded to legislators who ultimately disregarded their concerns:

> [The white women frequently believe that] all they have to do is give the government the facts and their problem will be taken care of. They become progressively disenchanted with what they view as the violation of their rights. . . . [Their] stories are stories of transformations: transformations into more self-confident and assertive women; into political activists who challenge the existing system and feel powerful in that challenge.[25]

In contrast, the African American and Native American women in Krauss's study started out with a mistrust of government, based on their experiences of racism, colonialism, and genocide. Although the majority of the participants in my study were white women, their levels of trust and fear of the government were clearly connected to their socioeconomic resources.

Even as women from middle-class and affluent backgrounds reported avoiding political activism, most described themselves as becoming empowered through the political process. Although the order of the questions in my interview—where I asked first how participants defined political activity and then whether and how they engaged in it—prompted some women to reassess their own definitions as we spoke (as is evident in the following quote), it is significant that only middle-class and affluent women reevaluated their initial answers in our conversations. For instance, Zora White, a college professor who had elected to parent full time at home when her first child was born, told me:

> I don't see myself as a political activist. It's like I try to stay as far away from political activity as possible—it really kinda turns my stomach. And if it weren't for something that was so near and dear to my heart, I wouldn't be doing this. . . . I only get as far as the letter writing, like I don't even wanna go talk to anybody about it because I just can't, I just don't like politicians at all, so I try to do things more on the outskirts, so I guess maybe you're stretching me to think about, maybe it is kinda political, some of the things I do, like, I'll talk to reporters or I'll do the educative piece with folks, trying to get the information out, and I guess that's political, ya know?[26]

Zora went on to explain how energized she felt when her children accompanied her to the legislature to watch testimony regarding a midwifery bill:

Just seeing the people sitting there on the floors and in the halls with all these babies, and moms with slings and the snacks . . . just saying, "Oh, this is so cool," that this could happen in Virginia. And just to see how overwhelmed the legislators were by it, ya know? It was new to them and-, it probably wasn't new to them, but they probably didn't want it to happen very often. And that really energized me to want to come back more.[27]

Although Zora tried *to stay as far away from political activity as possible*, she was ultimately *energized to come back* when she saw mothers' power to *overwhelm* legislators by bringing their children to the legislature.

Similarly, another homebirth mother, who lived in a wealthy suburban neighborhood and had recently begun training as a midwife when we spoke, explained:

See, what's weird is that I don't consider myself a political person at all. In fact, I'm very uncomfortable with politics. . . . I'm not a very political person. . . . I'm torn between attending those unattended births.[28] That was quite a statement, whether anyone knew I did it, that was kind of a statement, personally, but I guess, in the world, visibly, I've attended hearings, I did go to some before I [began training as a midwife and had more time], I did go talk with legislators . . . and write letters. I guess sitting in the hearings and bringing my three-and-a-half-year-old son along and nursing him in the front row, that was pretty empowering.[29]

Again, despite not considering herself *a very political person*, this aspiring midwife viewed the experience of nursing her son *in the front row* of the Virginia General Assembly as *pretty empowering*.

Likewise, Jackie Grayson, a self-described "stay-at-home mom" with multiple academic degrees who homeschools her children, explained:

I can't remember which vote it was . . . for the midwifery legislation. I was sitting in the room when they were doing the vote with the people that were on the committee and watching them watch us when they were about to say yes or no. I'm sitting there pregnant and there was someone else pregnant too and you're watching them look at us with the turmoil in their faces as to what to say. That time [the bill] passed in that level [but later got] rejected with the big guys. But it was wonderful, we all rejoiced, we were so thrilled . . . so excited. Just making that eye contact, sitting there very pregnant in the

only dress that fit me at that point . . . that was a really neat
experience.[30]

Even with the reluctance Jackie expressed earlier in our interview about engaging in political activity, she felt *so thrilled* and *so excited* to be a part of the
legislative process itself, particularly when she felt that her presence, *very
pregnant in the only dress that fit me at that point*, had persuaded lawmakers to
change their votes. This contrasted sharply with the fears that low-income
participants—who were often unable to afford the trips to Richmond to participate in the legislative process—expressed about the government's intervention in their lives.

During our interviews, low-income homebirthers frequently revealed
their fear of state repercussions, both for hiring midwives and participating
in—and including their children in—political activity to support midwives.
For instance, Dera Haviland, a single mother with what she described as "a
limited income," explained that one reason she was not more politically active
was her fear of arrest if she participated in political activity:

> My heart is a lot, is very much with nonviolent protesting and forms
> of protest that can be pretty in the front of things and I don't feel like
> I can do that given the fact that I'm raising two kids on my own and I
> don't have any extended network of family or friends that would,
> could raise them if something were to happen. . . . I don't know
> whether these are like latent beliefs from childhood, but I do get re-
> ally concerned about if I was to identify myself with pretty extreme
> activity that it could end up compromising being able to do things le-
> gitimately. And I don't know what's right.[31]

For Dera, who had few resources to tap into *if something were to happen*, participating in legislative efforts to support midwives seemed to be too great a
risk when it came to raising her children *legitimately*.

Although more affluent mothers were often quick to explain to me that
homebirth itself was *not* illegal, and that families who hired midwives were not
at risk themselves, low-income women still feared being incarcerated themselves, or losing their children to social service agencies over their decision to
homebirth or become involved in political efforts to support midwives. Elsa
Harden, for instance, worried about her neighbors' reactions to her decision to
homebirth as well as her family of eight living in a small three-bedroom house:

> I'm so worried because we don't vaccinate and we do use herbs and
> supplements and diet and we do homebirth. . . . I kept hearing things

from different states about people being arrested, kids taken away just because they had an unattended birth even though it was legal and everybody was fine. . . . We have neighbors around here who would just in a heartbeat call Social Services.[32]

Elsa was one of three women in my study who shared her experience of a planned, unassisted homebirth. She felt this option had become more common in Virginia, particularly after midwives started being investigated and arrested in the mid-to-late 1990s. Although no state or national data tease out the number of intentional unassisted births versus unintentional ones, many homebirthers believe that the number is rising. The proliferation of online resources dedicated to this subject in recent years has even prompted some to herald a "freebirth movement."[33] Although the participants in my study who chose unassisted births were from a range of socioeconomic backgrounds, much of the online discussion about unassisted homebirth suggests that it provides one option for women to "opt out" of the consumer-based medical model of birth, which, as one self-proclaimed "unassisted homebirth junkie" explained, "reinforces the materialism/consumerism our sick modern society is based on."[34] Nevertheless, this "nonconsumer" option still illuminates the socioeconomic differences in the ways in which women articulated their fears about giving birth in the home—whether alone, shared with close family members or friends, or attended by midwives.

In contrast to the more affluent homebirth mothers' confidence in the protection offered by the government and the legal system, low-income women repeatedly cited cases of children being removed from parental custody following unattended homebirths as well as underground midwife-attended homebirths. Although no comprehensive national data exist for these cases, and no one knew of any cases that occurred in Virginia, in 2002 I sent a query regarding this issue to a national Listserv of midwifery supporters and received personal stories of child custody cases related to homebirth in Iowa, Massachusetts, Pennsylvania, Rhode Island, and South Dakota. In these cases, state officials had often threatened parents with criminal charges of "child abuse" and "medical neglect," and children (both newborns and older children) were removed from their parents' custody for up to several weeks.[35] State officials often dropped the charges if parents would reveal their midwife's name. This evidence was then used against the midwife in ongoing or subsequent investigations.[36] It is also notable that the two quotes presented earlier by Paula and Evie, in which they linked the disrespect they had experienced in medical settings to their interactions with legislators, hint at their status as low-income homebirthers. None of the middle-class mothers I interviewed used metaphors, such as being *raped*, or that it was *obstetrics all over*, to link their experiences in the legislature to those they had had in hospitals. Likewise, although most homebirthers viewed their decision to hire underground midwives as a rejection of "mainstream consumerism," low-income women increasingly emphasized that their "choices" were often overscrutinized by the state.

Sociologist Chris Bobel, in her study *The Paradox of Natural Mothering*, discovered a similar pattern concerning women's assessment of risk among mothers committed to simple living and attachment parenting, a parenting philosophy that often includes extended breastfeeding, co-sleeping, and a commitment to natural foods and healthcare. All of the mothers in her study were white and predominately middle class, not unlike the broader demographic of "simple-livers."[37] Although many "natural mothers" believe that consumerism is one of America's most egregious social ills,[38] their class privilege ultimately influenced their willingness to take social risks, as well as to engage in political activity. Bobel explains:

> It is *because* they enjoy a secure economic status, solidified by their racial, educational, and class status, that they can afford to take the social risks involved in non-mainstream practices. In this sense, their privilege serves as a sort of safety net, protecting them from a nasty fall should they, for instance, be challenged for nursing their toddler in a public space or refusing conventional medical treatment for an illness. Being white and middle-class, they are less likely to come under attack. A poor woman of color spotted breastfeeding an older child could risk censure and certainly judgement.[39]

Although all of the homebirth mothers in my study were rightfully concerned about the public criticisms they received from medical officials in the legislature, the low-income women linked these concerns more directly to their fears of being identified as politically active.

"Homebirth *Is* a Political Act": Recasting Support for Midwives

Despite the persistent fears that many low-income mothers expressed, many also discussed alternative strategies in which they felt comfortable engaging—often on a more individual or community-based level than the more affluent homebirthers—in their support of midwives. For example, Val Coleman, a single mother who avoided political activism because she "keep[s] really busy trying to work to make money and support my kid," explained her "low-key" support of the homebirth mothers and midwives in her community:

> I've tried to support as many women in pregnancy and birth as possible and by providing teas, like herbal teas, emotional support, massage, those kinds of things, nothing really activist.[40]

Another homebirth mother, Gaia Riverton, who received prenatal care at a local hospital under their "indigent care" program, did not really consider herself politically active but told me this story:

> I think a lot of it is sharing with other women about my birth experience. Because, you know, even when you have a homebirth with [the local CNM], she asks you to go in to get preliminary tests done, so you're going into regular obstetricians' offices to get blood work or get a pelvic exam or whatever. And many, many times, I've been sitting for an hour or more in the waiting room, and there are, you know, twenty other pregnant women there, and some of them have got other little babies, and you start to talk to them, and it, inevitably you are talking about breastfeeding, or bottle-feeding, or where you're going to give birth. And it's been so interesting to talk with these women about, you know, what are their plans? You know, questioning that a little bit. I remember meeting one woman that had just never even considered breastfeeding, I mean, it just had never crossed her mind. She said, "But doesn't it hurt? But isn't it a pain in the butt?" And I just remember sitting down and giving her the number for the La Leche League and talking to her about my experience and it was just like, she had just never been exposed to that thinking before, and I think everything her doctor had been telling her and everything her friends had been telling her was that no one breastfeeds anymore. "They've got this stuff, you can just buy it at the store." . . . So, often I think, maybe I'll just come in two or three hours early for my appointment [laughs] and just talk with people. I've even thought about just setting up a table and passing out information! [laughs][41]

Gaia highlighted the political importance of talking to others, particularly those who were not aware of certain reproductive options or those who did not necessarily agree with her about homebirth. Engaging in conversation about personal choices in childbirth with fellow healthcare recipients became a public act for Gaia in the context of her obstetrician's waiting room: *I've even thought about just setting up a table and passing out information!*

Bobel's research with women who engaged in "natural mothering" suggests that many women committed to "voluntary simplicity" also "viewed their lives as strategic missions to effect social change."[42] This mirrored the sentiments of many women in my study across the socioeconomic spectrum, particularly in their commitment to homebirthing as a political act. What struck me as a socioeconomic difference in this commitment, however, was how low-income women frequently coupled their commitment to a politicized lifestyle, as well as their avoidance of legislative politics and direct grassroots organizing, with their hesitance regarding state intervention in their family life. As Dera, who shared her concerns about lack of family support regarding taking care of her children if she was arrested, explained:

> I'm raising two kids on my own and I've had not a lot of extra time or resources to put out into the world, so it becomes really important that everything I do becomes my political statement. It becomes my political statement that I don't take my kids to McDonald's. It becomes my political statement that I shop here, not there. It becomes my political statement, well it seems kind of goofy, but that's what I've turned all my political beliefs into. I do feel the need right now to kind of try to make my circle a little bigger, to become a little bit more articulate with policy makers and try to do something on that level, but I'm still pretty hesitant. And I definitely have a legacy with my parents being [immigrants]. My mother was very kind of wiggy about the way that if you didn't have security you wouldn't make it in the world. And definitely there is a political structure that certainly would condemn even my religious beliefs. I have certain fears and concerns of a political structure that really does condemn most of the choices I make. I'm certainly not going along with their program.[43]

Dera clearly politicizes her everyday consumer choices, *I don't take my kids to McDonald's* and *I shop here, not there*, in the same way many of the middle-class women in Bobel's study did. But as a daughter of Lithuanian immigrants to the United States who was raising two children alone on an annual income of approximately $10,000, she expressed different concerns about the state than her middle-class counterparts.

Like Dera, and in contrast to the visible grassroots organizers who served on the boards of emerging nonprofit organizations and political action committees and those who were active on statewide Listservs to unite midwifery supporters, most low-income women did not identify as members of grassroots organizations to support midwives. Yet many low-income midwifery supporters also felt that the act of having a homebirth was a way in which *all* homebirthers were politically active. Terri Jacobs, who lived in a rural community with no running water or electricity, wrote in a rare post to a grassroots organizing Listserv, "Having a homebirth makes you a political creature by default, like-it-or-not."[44] Evie, who spoke about being disrespected by legislators and obstetricians and was one of the few low-income homebirth mothers I interviewed who had become active in state-wide organizing efforts and in the legislature, explained, "I just don't get up into what's going on in Washington [politically] because I'm to the point where everything I see, the lines between my everyday life and every breath is political and every woman's life is a statement."[45] At times, however, the broader definitions of "political activity" articulated by low-income homebirthers put them at odds with middle-class organizers who sought more specifically to persuade legislators to change laws that restricted their access to midwives.

For example, Crystal Roberts, a prominent organizer who was instrumental in e-mail campaigns to persuade homebirth mothers from around the state to travel to Richmond to attend the debates over midwifery bills, chided fellow homebirthers for participating in the *political act* of having a homebirth but not becoming politically active in other ways:

> So, any one of you who had [a homebirth]—whether it was [with] a CNM, a direct-entry midwife, or by yourself—it was a political act. And I think that the midwives really suffer [when they] try to keep that barrier between their clients and that political act by trying-, not making those consumers aware of [the political nature of their homebirths] and be[coming] responsible for that.[46]

Unfortunately, low-income women were not always welcome in their attempts to join middle-class homebirthers to advocate for midwives in the legislature or with medical officials, as I discuss further in Chapter 6. Moreover, the risks they incurred made their "everyday" political acts directed at broad social change (such as talking to other mothers about the benefits of breastfeeding or avoiding the consumerism of McDonald's) far less risky than exposing themselves in overtly "political" arenas.

Despite the fact that *most* homebirth mothers did not characterize their actions to support midwives as political, the stakes were invariably higher for low-income women. While middle-class and affluent women could use their political skills and influence in the legislative arena, low-income women were frequently absent from such legislative discussions.[47] Within this context, identification as consumers rather than political actors became compelling for many middle-class midwifery supporters who felt empowered by their ability to highlight their economic power in the face of the medical establishment's efforts to discredit them. This did not seem to be a viable option for low-income women, however, who instead emphasized their feelings of disempowerment by doctors and their fears of persecution by the government. These women felt that their right to live and mother as they chose could be taken away. These different experiences and concerns are posing challenging new dilemmas for organizers as they attempt to draw together homebirth mothers from diverse socioeconomic backgrounds in their struggle for access to midwives.

6

Divisive Strategies

Struggles for Reproductive Rights
under Neoliberalism

Corporate capitalism has redefined citizens as consumers—
and global markets replace commitments to economic,
social, and racial equality.
—CHANDRA TALPADE MOHANTY,
FEMINISM WITHOUT BORDERS

A s midwives became increasingly involved in legislative efforts to legalize their practice in Virginia, more and more of their supporters began to characterize their struggle as one for "consumer rights" within
the legislature and grassroots organizing efforts. Although natural childbirth
proponents had first adopted a consumer identity to advocate against medicalized childbirth in the 1960s and 1970s, contemporary homebirthers' attempts to claim *rights* as consumers stem from a much longer history of political and economic shifts toward neoliberalism in the United States—and
throughout much of the world—a history that has prioritized consumer rights
over citizens' rights. It is important to remember, however, that the socioeconomic inequalities that these recent shifts have exacerbated cannot be
attributed solely to the advent of neoliberalism.[1] Rather, they appear along
familiar fault lines of racialized and class-based divisions within the United
States. Thus this chapter begins with a brief overview of the shifting concept
of "rights" in the twentieth century, specifically, who has had and who has
laid claim to particular rights at different points in U.S. history. I argue that
claims to "the right to choose," which intensified during struggles for women's
rights in the 1960s and 1970s, have now shifted toward a more singular focus
on "consumer rights" under neoliberalism, and that this has potentially dire
consequences for the future of reproductive rights more broadly.

During my initial interviews with midwifery supporters in 2000 and 2001,
almost all participants—regardless of their political or religious affiliations—
referred to their "right to choose" midwives as something that was being denied

to them by the state. In addition, approximately one-third of the participants used the term "consumer" specifically to describe themselves and/or other midwifery supporters, often correcting my reference to them as "political advocates," "activists," or "grassroots organizers." Several also corrected my reference to the movement for midwifery as a group of "people," "individuals," or "mothers," preferring to highlight their—and others'—political participation as consumers. Homebirthers often framed their identity as "consumers" as a strategy to differentiate themselves from the midwives who were advocating for their professional needs and as a convenient term to mobilize women from a broad range of political and religious constituencies. Notably, however, most of those who used the term "consumer" in our interviews reported annual household income levels of more than $50,000 a year. Most were also older than childbearing age or not planning to have any more children, implying that putting themselves in the political category "consumer" was less a descriptive term than it was a strategic tactic to make use of the state's terminology (and values) to attain their political objectives.

My discussion of access to midwifery becoming characterized as a "consumer's right" becomes additionally complex in the context of recent legislative successes for midwifery advocates in Virginia and other states. Through their political victories, it becomes clear that "consumer rights" rhetoric is convincing to the state officials who decide whether to open up the market of reproductive services to midwives. For those pursuing midwife licensure, then, arguing for the "consumer's right" to choose a birthcare practitioner remains an essential and a strategic use of market-based terminology. What I question, however, is how historically uneven access to reproductive healthcare services will ultimately play out for the socioeconomically diverse families who currently seek access to midwifery care in areas such as Virginia. My interviews with low-income homebirthers revealed serious concerns about identifying access to midwives as a "consumer's right" and the differential impact that such strategies could have on women's ability to choose from a broad range of reproductive options into the twenty-first century.

Claiming Rights in the United States: A Brief Overview

Political and social understandings of "citizens' rights" in the United States changed substantially in the twentieth century. The *idea* of rights for U.S. citizens is, of course, nothing new. The Declaration of Independence stated in 1776, "We hold these truths to be self-evident, that all men are created equal, that they are endowed by their Creator with certain unalienable

Rights, that among these are Life, Liberty and the pursuit of Happiness."[2] However, the government has not evenly awarded the rights and privileges associated with citizenship. Among other rights initially accorded only to white male citizens, women and minorities were notably excluded from voting—a privilege widely touted as one of the most important rights for citizens in a democracy. By the early twentieth century, however, these groups had collectively struggled for—and won—voting rights (even though it took the Voting Rights Act of 1965 to abolish the discriminatory practices that kept African Americans from voting freely). Yet as historian Sara Evans has argued, the extension of suffrage beyond white men in the United States created fundamental changes to the concept of citizenship. In her work on women's suffrage, she wrote:

> With one stroke the Nineteenth Amendment enfolded women into a particular version of the American political heritage, defining citizenship as a relationship between the individual and the state, whose key expression was the act of voting. To win this right, women had to organize together, to act as a group. But the right itself undermined collectivity. . . . Many of the leaders of the suffrage movement believed that once women had the right to vote they would, as individuals, express . . . female values through the electoral process and there would be no more need for collective organization. But these "female values" really represented the politicized domesticity of middle-class women with its associated prejudices towards blacks, immigrants and the working class.[3]

Thus in 1920, after women's initial victory of suffrage, several growing concerns for proponents of women's rights became clear. First, women had not attained full equality with men—economically, socially, or politically—with merely the right to vote alongside them. Although suffragists had initially hoped that women would join together through their voting power to make other legal changes, this collective power did not materialize. Recall, for instance, the repeal of the Sheppard-Towner Maternal and Infant Health Act in 1929, discussed in Chapter 1, after male politicians became aware that women were not voting as a unified collective. Second, as also evident in the differential effects that the Sheppard-Towner Act had on white and minority women (not to mention midwives), universal equality for *all* women had not been achieved through suffrage alone. Women's rights—to equal pay, educational equity and, perhaps still most controversially, reproductive freedom—continued to be stratified by their race, nationality, and class. Although the Civil Rights Act of 1964 made broad gains for African Americans, minority women in the 1960s still found that their issues of concern were largely ignored both within male-led civil rights organizations and primarily white feminist groups.[4]

As women struggled to address these contradictions, the "second wave" of the women's movement emerged during the 1960s and encouraged political activism that focused on the social, as well as the legal, inequities that women continued to face after they won the right to vote. While I agree with the feminist scholars who have argued that this was not, in fact, a "new" women's movement but rather a resurgence of activism with roots in the work of suffragists from the early twentieth century,[5] what *was* new was the way in which feminists began to make claims to rights. Claims to "human rights," for example, which became common after the phrase appeared in the United Nations Charter in 1945, were particularly compelling for feminists who sought to address issues of broad concern to women throughout the world, such as violence against women and access to reproductive healthcare. As cultural theorist Inderpal Grewal has argued, the concept of human rights, that "all human beings are born free and equal in dignity and rights,"[6] quickly became "almost the only way to address issues of social justice, oppression, and inequality" throughout the world.[7] This emphasis on individual rights opened up new possibilities for different constituencies to pursue claims to rights in the courts— which eventually allowed for clashes between competing individual rights, such as the "right to life" of the unborn and women's "right to choose" reproductive health services, including contraception and abortion.[8]

Understanding what led to the coupling of reproductive rights with human rights in the United States, however, requires a closer look at several important legal cases that occurred during the mid-twentieth century. In 1942, as human rights issues were initially gaining worldwide currency before being codified in the UN Charter in 1945, the U.S. Supreme Court issued a key decision in *Skinner v. Oklahoma* about compulsory contraception that historian Rickie Solinger has argued "tied reproduction itself to human rights [and] clearly began to define a concept of *reproductive rights.*"[9] Earlier legal and legislative decisions in the United States had upheld forced sterilization of those deemed "unfit" by state and local governments. A particularly sobering example is Carrie Buck, a poor young woman from Charlottesville, Virginia, who was labeled "feebleminded" and sentenced to compulsory sterilization after having a child out of wedlock.[10] Her case, *Buck v. Bell*, ultimately went to the U.S. Supreme Court, in 1927, where Virginia's sterilization laws were upheld as constitutional, and Justice Oliver Wendell Holmes issued the infamous declaration (referring to Buck, her mother, and her newborn) "three generations of imbeciles are enough."[11] Ethnic studies scholar Nancy Ordover has argued that this case was "part of a deliberate and determined effort to situate women as the primary candidates for sterilization" during the early 1900s.[12] In 1942, however, in the *Skinner v. Oklahoma* case, Jack T. Skinner, a white man convicted of stealing chickens, was originally sentenced to sterilization for his crime under Oklahoma's sterilization laws, but the Supreme Court ruled that forced sterilization was "an encroachment on basic liberty."[13] Although it is perhaps ironic that the first association of "reproduction" and "rights" in U.S. law was tied to a white man (though not terribly surprising, given the history of rights development in the United States, where many rights have initially been accorded to white propertied men and then extended), this decision was significant to women's ability to claim reproductive rights "as a keystone of their citizenship status" during the rest of the twentieth century.[14]

It is also notable that this initial articulation of reproductive rights centered around a case regarding compulsory sterilization, not—as many would come to associate reproductive rights later in the twentieth century—around abortion. Sociologist Kristin Luker has traced the first claims to abortion specifically as a right to 1961, when women emerged as a "self-conscious interest group," different than the primarily professional interests expressed on the issue prior to that time.[15] A central event that solidified emerging feminist arguments that women should have the *right* to make reproductive choices was the case of Sherri Finkbine in 1962. Finkbine was a married mother of four who lived in a suburb of Phoenix, Arizona. When she was pregnant with her fifth child, she was prescribed medication for morning sickness that she later learned contained thalidomide, a drug that had recently been shown to cause extensive fetal abnormalities, such as a baby being born without arms or legs and with severe heart problems. Finkbine's doctor advised her to have a "therapeutic abortion" (the only kind of abortion legal at that time, when a mother's health was thought to be at risk). However, when hospital administrators refused and Finkbine eventually flew to Sweden to obtain a legal abortion, a public debate about her case was initiated throughout the United States. Although Finkbine did not argue for abortion *as a right*, her public statements suggested that "a woman—especially a well-dressed, attractive, middle-class, married woman, a mother of four, like herself—could justifiably make a choice about a pregnancy that had already taken hold."[16]

Finkbine's case became symbolic for the growing feminist movement, and it opened up new possibilities for women's organizing, not only for the right to obtain a legal abortion but also for the right to contraception. Thus women's activism for reproductive rights as a "women's rights" issue intensified over the 1960s and into the early 1970s. In 1965, the Supreme Court invalidated a Connecticut law from 1879, which prohibited the use of contraceptives, in *Griswold v. Connecticut* on the grounds that it violated the "right to marital privacy."[17] The right to contraceptives, then, was initially available only to married couples. In 1972, this "right to privacy" was extended in *Eisenstadt v. Baird*, when the Supreme Court struck down a Massachusetts law prohibiting the distribution of contraceptives to unmarried people, ruling that it violated the Equal Protection Clause of the U.S. Constitution.[18] The surge of women's activism that accompanied these decisions culminated in the *Roe v. Wade* Supreme Court decision in 1973, which legalized abortion in the United States.[19] As Luker has explained in *Abortion and the Politics of Motherhood*, however, this decision came largely as a surprise to nonprofessional opponents of abortion at the time. Thus 1973 inaugurated the emergence of the right-to-life movement, which argued that "personhood is a 'natural,' inborn, and inherited right," and that individualized rights should extend to the unborn, an "interest group" that, unlike women, could not speak for themselves.[20] Arguments over when a fetus becomes a person, and should thus be accorded human rights, have remained under contentious debate to the present day.

In *Beggars and Choosers*, Solinger has argued that the notion of reproductive rights as human rights inaugurated the "era of choice" during the 1960s and 1970s, which ultimately defined some groups as "good" choice makers and others as "bad."[21] Not unlike the experience of homebirth mothers in the legislature, discussed in Chapter 4, the resulting conundrum has forced all women—especially those who must make decisions about childbirth or mothering practices—to find new ways to demonstrate to policy makers their respectability as "good" choice makers. Notably, neoliberal political and economic shifts have reinforced and intensified ideas about "good" citizenship being actualized through one's choices as a consumer within the market economy. Although political scientists and historians have demonstrated that the "citizen as consumer was a growing political presence," by the early twentieth century, when "the growth of large retail stores such as department stores, chain stores, and mail-order businesses also encouraged Americans to think and act politically as consumers,"[22] broad claims to "consumer rights" were not initially associated with citizens' rights *to consume* goods and resources but rather struggles for consumer safety and protection from corporate monopolies.[23] A familiar example that coincided with the natural childbirth movement during the 1960s and 1970s was the group "Nader's Raiders," led by consumer advocate Ralph Nader, who investigated safety concerns for "citizen-consumers."[24] The shift toward recognizing each citizen's right to consume goods and services came with the struggle for "consumer choice" during the 1960s and 1970s during the civil rights movement (for access to markets that had formerly been denied to African Americans) and among feminists (for the "right to choose" abortion and contraception).[25] Yet it was the advent of neoliberalism in the 1980s and 1990s that brought with it a shift toward thinking about citizens' rights as those that could—and should—be determined *by* the market. In fact, governmental control over citizens' rights became suspect, a potential threat to individual choices. Previous notions of the government's role as a guarantor of citizens' rights were eclipsed by the idea that individual rights to free choice were best achieved through open markets.

Yet despite the rhetoric of universal rights for all citizens under neoliberalism, access to basic rights are denied to those who do not or can not consume appropriately.[26] As political theorist Barbara Cruikshank summarizes: "We have different kinds citizens who are recognized not for what they do or what they have been made into but for what they lack."[27] With the growing influence of neoliberal ideology on public policy decisions since the 1980s, activists have been forced to lay claim to rights not as citizens but, rather, as consumers of goods and services. As historian Alice Kessler-Harris has explained, "In modern democratic societies prevailing beliefs in the sanctity of the market make access to it the only practical route to empowerment as citizens."[28]

For reproductive rights advocates, the draw of "consumer rights" has been particularly compelling, as a woman's "right to choose" can easily be extended to her choices within the growing market of reproductive healthcare options. Yet as I indicated earlier, the allure of "consumer rights" creates new problems for activists who are committed to organizing for the rights of *all* women. Women only have the privilege to make choices within the marketplace of reproductive options if they have the resources to enter it to begin with. Promoting the rights only of the individual consumer, then, ultimately reiterates exclusions that have historically plagued feminist efforts to promote rights for all women. As Solinger has noted regarding feminists' initial adoption of the "right to choose" in the 1970s, "our Constitution does not, of course, guarantee anyone the *right* to enter the marketplace of reproductive (or any other) options."[29] As I demonstrate later, using the push for midwives in Virginia as one example, these shifting definitions of "rights" and "citizenship" are having profound effects on contemporary struggles for reproductive rights.

Midwifery Consumers and the "Right to Choose"

At the first midwifery advocacy meeting I attended in Virginia in 1999, organizers identified themselves explicitly as midwifery "consumers," despite the fact that most were not actively seeking the care of midwives. The facilitator of the Virginia Midwifery Coalition (VMC) meeting, a group that brought together leaders from midwifery and homebirth support groups from throughout the state, asked participants to brainstorm regarding the composition of

Virginia's "midwifery community." She categorized participants' responses into three levels, which she wrote on a nearby flipchart:

1. those who were actively participating in VMC
2. those who would likely participate in VMC and the broader movement for midwifery
3 those who would be affected by the actions of VMC

The first two categories could include what social movement theorists have called "potential beneficiaries," those who would or could benefit from the successes of the group, and "conscience constituents," those who are direct supporters of an organization but do not stand to benefit directly from the accomplishment of its goals.[30] Many of those in attendance at the VMC's meeting were, in fact, conscience constituents. Although most were mothers who had had their children at home, not midwives themselves, who were frequently unable to attend organizational meetings because of their twenty-four hour "on-call" commitment to the pregnant women in their care elsewhere in the state, the majority of those mothers did not plan to have additional children. Many explained that their interest in supporting midwives stemmed from their desire to make midwives available to *all* women and families in Virginia.

Thus it was significant when the participants identified "consumers," those who would benefit from legal access to midwives, in both the first and second tiers as members or potential members of the midwifery movement, but not in the third tier: those affected by the VMC's efforts to increase legal access to midwives. Instead, "all citizens" were identified in the third category as those who would be affected by, but not involved in, midwifery advocacy. What is notable about this delineation is that midwifery supporters characterized their political participation in the VMC and "the broader movement for midwifery" through their role as consumers of midwifery services rather than as interested citizens who were political advocates for midwives or activists who represented women deserving of reproductive rights as citizens. "All citizens" were instead placed in a depoliticized category, those who would be affected by the (political) actions of consumers. As noted earlier, political struggles for rights based on an individual's ability to consume them have significantly different implications than broader struggles for rights that affect "all citizens." Identifying themselves as consumers of midwifery services—despite the fact that the majority of those present did not plan to have additional children— highlighted the ways in which recent neoliberal political shifts have changed the terms of contemporary activists' efforts.

During my subsequent fieldwork and interviews, midwifery supporters frequently drew attention to their legitimacy as consumers to make claims to the right to have a homebirth with the practitioner of their choice. One long-time midwifery supporter, Thomas Danforth, whose children and grandchildren were born at home, was among the first to suggest that mothers, as consumers of childbirth services, deserved full rights within the Commonwealth of Virginia.

> The state is depriving its citizens (consumers) of rightful access to safe and affordable maternity care by prohibiting [direct-entry] midwifery. As "consumers," you and your child are being exposed to damages (health and economic) due to the fact that [direct-entry] midwifery is prohibited.[31]

Though Thomas restricted his use of *consumers* in parentheses and then in quotes, his acknowledgment of the state's understanding of citizens as consumers is important because the consumer status of the homebirther is characterized as a political status. Thus Thomas suggests that as consumers, rather than as mothers or activists or citizens, both women and children are at risk of *being exposed to damages (both health and economic)* because of the state's prohibition of DEMs.

During their lobbying efforts, homebirth mothers also identified themselves to lawmakers as consumers, frequently as a way to emphasize the precarious legal and economic situation of homebirth mothers in Virginia in relation to reproductive healthcare providers. Recall Ellen Hamblet's testimony to legislators, that "consumers are caught in the middle of poor relations between doctors and midwives."[32] Many organizers felt that the term "consumer" was an important means by which to differentiate themselves from birthcare practitioners who had professional stakes in the legislation at hand. As Fern Jackson, a homebirth mother who had spoken with legislators both privately and publicly in support of midwives, explained:

> One problem we've had in Richmond is it really doesn't make sense when you look at the way their [the legislative] system is created, it really does not make sense for a consumer group to be doing the kind of advocacy work that we're [doing]. . . . They assume that we're all midwives, because why would somebody who's not a midwife be talking about licensure for midwives? That's a professional thing to do, not a consumer thing to do.[33]

Fern further explained her rights within the context of the U.S. Constitution. She felt that as a *reasonable citizen*, the state should preserve her right to hire a midwife.

I think pretty highly of myself as being very well educated, very concerned about my children and their health and well-being, very well
informed, the idea that I could go and do all that research and make
my decision, okay, this is what is best for me and for my family, and
then to have the state tell me, "No, you can't make that decision because you can't hire a midwife for homebirth." "We think that homebirth is too dangerous," which has been their stated objection. . . . It's
so anti-American, it's anti-everything this country stands for and I am
pretty committed to the kind of ideals that the country stands for. . . .
And I don't think I can point to a specific place where it [the Consti-
tution] says it, but it certainly implies in there that reasonable citizens
should be able to do their own research and make their own decisions
about something like who they want to hire, where they want to give
birth to their baby. And the state has no business in standing in the
way of that. That's not why states were founded or constructed to ba-
sically, ya know, to protect the monopoly on healthcare by the medical system.[34]

Although, as discussed earlier, the U.S. Constitution does not guarantee
women the right to enter the marketplace of reproductive options, Fern makes
the argument that the state *should* grant *reasonable citizens* the right to choose
both where and with whom they give birth. To do otherwise, she contends, is
anti-American, particularly when it is done in a state effort *to protect the monopoly on healthcare by the medical system*. Like many midwifery advocates, Fern
hoped that their local movement would contribute to broader resistance to
mainstream, increasingly commercialized types of childbirth under the biomedical model. Accordingly, she and others felt midwifery advocates should
use the term "consumer" to make important distinctions between those who
hire midwives and those who seek licensure *as* midwives.

In contrast, physicians almost exclusively used the term "patient" to describe those seeking reproductive healthcare. Most midwives and homebirth
mothers, however, avoided the term "patient," which they felt indicated illness,
as well as a denial of the woman's agency in the childbirth process. Many
opted for the term "client" to describe those who sought midwives' services to
acknowledge their healthy status as pregnant women making active choices
about their reproductive care. But when midwives referred to their clients *as
political actors*, they did so largely as "consumers." As one busy midwife explained, "I think it has to be consumer efforts, and I think the consumers
[have to be the ones to support legislation for midwives] because . . . most
[midwives] are employed, and how can they be employed at the same time that
they are [spending their time advocating for legislation]?"[35]

Some midwives—in my study and more broadly—have been more ambivalent about referring to the women in their care as "consumers." In her study of Canadian midwives in Ontario, for example, anthropologist Margaret MacDonald explained:

> When clients approach [midwifery] as just another consumer choice, it feels to some midwives like a decontextualized understanding and use of midwifery. I have heard it called "midwifery a la mode" or the "midwifery spritzer." . . . Midwives would like their clients to understand midwifery not simply as a new consumer option but as the culmination of a significant social and political movement that challenged the status quo.[36]

Similarly, sociologist Ivy Lynn Bourgeault's work with midwives and their supporters in Ontario revealed that midwives and mothers often found terms such as "caregiver" and "client" insufficient to describe the "more egalitarian, friendship-oriented relationship" between midwives and the families in their care.[37] Most midwives in my study expressed similar concerns about the importance of acknowledging the depth of their relationship with the women in their care, but many midwives who served primarily a middle-class clientele had also incorporated the term "consumer" into their language, as noted earlier. Midwives who served low-income homebirthers seemed less certain, as the following quote from a midwife who was practicing underground in an impoverished community illustrates:

> We're saying this is a consumer issue. . . . That word is used, that's the commonly used word, "consumer." . . . The people who can organize on the, I'm going to use the word consumer because I don't know what other word to use, but the people who are seeking access to this care [from all socioeconomic backgrounds], know what they want.[38]

By stumbling over and questioning the term "consumer"—*I'm going to use the word consumer because I don't know what other word to use*—this midwife highlights how limited this term is when referring to the low-income women she serves and, at the same time, its clear salience to broader organizing efforts.

I observed a similar difference regarding the socioeconomic circumstances of participants in the various ways that homebirth mothers used the popular feminist slogan "a woman's right to choose" to justify why they should have access to midwives. It is also significant that study participants who used this phrase came from diverse political and religious backgrounds. Zora White, for instance, introduced in Chapter 5, who was a stay-at-home mom after leaving her position as a college professor, described herself as a feminist and a Democrat. Not surprisingly, as a feminist committed to women's "right to choose," she explained: "[Midwifery is] a women's right-to-choose issue, about empowering women instead of shutting them up. . . . I really really do see it as an issue of feminism, probably more than anything else."[39] In contrast, Anna Turner, who was also a stay-at-home mother following her career in the military, described herself as a "conservative Christian homebirther." She also explained her support of midwifery in the context of "choice," albeit more ambivalently:

> I feel like my choices have just been dwindled away. It affects me, it affects my family. It's weird though, here I'm saying I'm a Christian and I support this [midwifery] and I don't like abortion, and I notice people talk about choice and being able to choose. And I just want to differentiate between [them]. I believe that life is a gift of God and that's something I believe that life and death should be with God. So, I just wanted to mention that too, instead of, because I'm talking about choice, you know, I want to choose my midwife. . . . Maybe I need another word instead of choice.[40]

Nonetheless, the language of choice has remained powerful for homebirthers, even for religiously and politically conservative ones. As another conservative homebirther wrote to a Listserv supporting midwifery legislation:

> Isn't it amazing that we live in a country that gives a woman the right over her body, the right to abuse it with alcohol, tobacco and drugs. We have the right to pierce our bodies and to wear little clothing out in public taunting men. Women have the right to abort a healthy baby, even those that are viable outside the womb. We do not, oddly, have the right to choose with whom we give birth nor where we give birth without being criticized, ridiculed, persecuted or prosecuted. How peculiar![41]

Although conservative homebirthers were not allied with broader feminist efforts for women's right to legally access to abortion and (in most cases) contraception, their arguments mimicked the popular feminist language of reproductive rights: women should *have the right to choose* a midwife.

Cindy Newton, the midwifery advocate introduced in Chapter 5 who testified before legislators as a "consumer advocate," described an even broader commitment to a woman's right to choose regarding reproductive health. As well as advocating for midwives, Cindy explained:

I want to be able to be fair to the women that want even maybe the scheduled Cesarean, women who are having trouble getting their Cesarean scheduled because it is an elective scheduled Cesarean for them. I believe that if those women are educated, and know the risks, and know what they are doing, and it fits in with their lifestyle, and that's what they want to do, and they may have other issues of why they don't want a vaginal birth, then I think that's their right also. I feel very strongly that birth is a very individual thing and that you need to be able to do it the way it feels right for you, not the way it feels right to some other person.[42]

Even though Cindy differs from most other midwifery advocates in her support of women who choose elective Cesarean sections, she emphasizes that mothers, as consumers of childbirth services, should have both the right and ability to *do what feels right for [them]*. Although Cindy identified herself as a "pro-life Republican," she felt that it was her duty to "represent the consumers" to legislators considering any issue that affected reproductive rights for women *during* childbirth.

Understanding themselves as consumers has also made the issue of choice among homebirth mothers—and, more to the point, who has reproductive healthcare choices—more complicated. Although many contemporary U.S. citizens view choice "as the key right of American identity: we want the ability to choose,"[43] feminist scholars have also reminded us that "choice" and the ability to "consume" reproductive rights and services mean different things to different women due to their cultural and economic circumstances. Notably, all of the mothers cited earlier who identified access to midwifery as a woman's right to choose—whether their views were liberal or conservative—had family incomes well above the median for their counties. Research on stratified reproduction demonstrates how choices are always made within the context of larger institutional structures, ideological messages, and financial limitations.[44] As anthropologist Rayna Rapp has explained in her study of women's choices about whether or not to have amniocentesis—a prenatal test for genetic abnormalities, such as Down's syndrome, that has a risk of miscarriage—it was the "scientifically confident middle-class women who felt empowered to make a decision 'against the grain,'" to choose to forgo the procedure, whereas clinic patients were more likely to refuse the test indirectly by being a "no-show" for one or more of their scheduled appointments.[45] Thus although those in Rapp's study who chose to forgo amniocentesis ultimately made the same decision, the women did so for different reasons and in different ways, and their "choices" were made in the context of both their economic and social relationship to medical institutions.

Similarly, the ways in which homebirth mothers in my study experienced reproductive choices frequently influenced their strategies for supporting midwives and guaranteeing women's ability to homebirth. Prior to 2005 legislation that licensed CPMs in Virginia, for instance, several participants suggested that decriminalizing the practice of DEMs, in lieu of licensing particular practitioners, would allow them to make such individualized choices. Although I do not wish to imply that support for particular pieces of legislation among midwifery supporters fell neatly along class lines, which it did not, many participants who expressed the ability to choose among reproductive healthcare service providers also believed that a "free" market would ensure that "consumers" would receive the best care available. Homebirth mother Tara Mason, who lived in a wealthy rural community, explained:

> I really have mixed feelings about it [licensure]. In Virginia, since we have a law banning DEMs, then getting them legalized again would definitely increase the access to them, but it will certainly include certain regulations that are probably going to be more restrictive than is necessary. One midwife I know, with more breech birth experience than most OBs [obstetricians], says up to 25 percent of her clients she would have to transfer out to an OB if she were to follow the restrictions most CNMs and CPMs have to abide by. Licensure is nice for governments to recognize those midwives that meet the level of training they want them to have, but shouldn't be necessary for all midwives. Consumers should be able to choose who they want at their births. . . . It would be best if the state would just register midwives, but let them practice within their own scope, and let them be regulated by other midwives and the consumers who would hire them.[46]

Ultimately, Tara's concern was that state regulation would restrict local midwives' practices and thus legislation would limit, rather than expand, *consumer* choices.

Similarly, Nelly Vicars, a homebirth mother who had been born at home herself and now lived in a wealthy suburban neighborhood, explained how she saw the free market and consumer education as a solution to the quandary over midwifery legislation:

> I don't think they should be licensed or regulated. . . . I'm really in favor of a free market. Say my neighbor across the street is a midwife and she's delivering babies, and I really haven't heard good things about her and if she's doing these cases that are just botched she's obviously going to go out of business because no one is going to go to her.

> I think it's the responsibility of the consumer to educate themselves and say: "What do I want to look for?" and "What kind of references does she have?" and those kinds of things. That would totally take care of regulating and licensure of them. They wouldn't need to be strictly regulated. So, I'd like to see the free market kind of take it over.[47]

One of the primary arguments against homebirth and midwifery from both state and medical officials is that it is the government's duty to "protect" mothers and babies—as indicated in physicians' legislative testimony in Chapter 4—from having to make such choices. Although these officials frequently debated whether homebirthers, such as Nelly, should be qualified to make informed decisions about their healthcare, most homebirthers believed that the research they had done—either by reading published material on safety in childbirth or through consultations with other homebirthers—was sufficient. For Nelly, choice was understood not only as an opportunity for the consumer but also as a *responsibility*.

Although the idea of a free market, under which individuals ultimately choose the best birth attendants for themselves, has been compelling for many midwifery supporters, Sheryl Ruzek reminds us that a consumer model often "appeals to people who are affluent because an unspoken assumption is that those who have more will get 'the best.' The assumption elevates choice to an ultimate value, an entitlement, something to be protected against erosion."[48] Thus while the consumer model offered some midwifery advocates a useful metaphor to describe themselves as citizens, it did not speak to the experiences of women who have restricted options for birthcare.

Indeed, many low-income women also favored decriminalization regarding the regulation and licensure of midwives but, like the women in Rapp's study of amniocentesis, their reasons for doing so were significantly different. Many were concerned that the government would punish them for seeking out local midwives who were not licensed by the state if others could be licensed. As discussed in the previous chapter, Val Coleman, the single mother who described her "low-key" support of other homebirth mothers by providing herbals teas, massage, and emotional support, explained:

> I just want to be completely anonymous and invisible, and do my thing, and live my truth, and not be bothered because I'm really a good person and I want to do things the way I think I want to do them, and that's not always politically correct or legal.[49]

Likewise, Nancy Davis, a single mother from a rural community whose income was just below the federal poverty line, emphasized that her individual lifestyle choices should not fall under government purview, and thus she made her childbirth choices accordingly:

> I never questioned–, I didn't want to ask somebody if it was okay for me to have my baby the way I wanted. There was no question for me. It was kind of actually more of a setting apart of me and the government because it's like, okay, I know that we disagree on this, and am I going to give you all my power? No. I'm going to do it my way and know that it's right, and it is. That's what I did.[50]

Both Val and Nancy felt that it was more important to be *anonymous and invisible* in their childbirth choices than to avoid confrontation with legal authorities.

Whereas the more affluent participants in my study often felt it was their *right* to have choices and control in their childbirth experience,[51] many low-income participants indicated an *interest* in choices regarding their birthcare but also a dependence on midwives as a low-cost childbirth option. In some cases, local low-cost midwifery services afforded those who did not have the option of consuming mainstream hospital childbirth services the opportunity to draw on an alternative form of birthcare (albeit in an underground economy at the time of my interviews). Kevin Rogers, a father whose three children were born at home, assisted by community midwives, explained that restricted economic resources encouraged his family to make the "choice" to hire a local underground midwife:

> We're not like the normal midwife consumers or clients. . . . It's also a financial issue with midwifery, in choosing midwifery too. We didn't have health insurance and didn't have income to be able to afford a hospital birth, couldn't figure out a way to do it. It was really dragging us down, and midwives were very reasonable.[52]

In this sense, Kevin set his family apart from what he considered—or perhaps what he thought I, as a middle-class researcher, considered—*normal midwife consumers or clients* who could afford *health insurance* and extensive childbirth options, including *hospital birth*. Instead, Kevin and his wife Sara described the reciprocal economic relationship that they had developed with their community midwives:

> SARA: Our midwives are local, our friends, and I don't know, we have this feeling or this belief that we look out for them, like they did something for us that we could never repay no matter if it's money

or if it's whatever. . . . They're in our thoughts as far as when we
have extra stuff—it could be money or if it's food. . . . It's the
belief that they're part of our community and we will always look
out for them.

KEVIN: We fix their cars, do all kinds of crazy stuff for them. . . . Bad
luck, not taking care of the midwife.[53]

Thus Sara and Kevin considered their relationship with their midwives not as
a *consumer* or *client* but as a *friend* and *part of our community*. Their lack of
identification with other *normal midwifery consumers or clients* becomes even
clearer when we consider the lengths some low-income women had to go to
access quality birthcare.

Many of the low-income homebirthers I interviewed who did not have
health insurance mentioned the option of going to public clinics for their
birthcare, but they also cited their own or other community members' experiences of being disrespected in free medical clinics to explain why they pre
ferred to seek community-based midwives, who frequently offered sliding
scale or barter options for payment. Paula Queen, who in the previous chapter described her experience in the hospital and with legislators as being
"raped," initially identified herself to me as "middle class." Yet she shared her
remarkable story of finding a midwife earlier in her life when she could not
afford to go to the hospital:

I didn't have a lot of money, I wouldn't say I was poor, but I was still
paying off hospital bills for [my last baby], and when I was pregnant, I
didn't have the money to go to the hospital—well I did, but I didn't feel
it was God's will for me to be in debt like that. So . . . I called
around—I actually called the state—I called all the health departments looking for midwives. They were like, "We used to have one!"
And then I called the state: "Well, we have a list. If you send us thirty-
five dollars, we'll give you a list of certified midwives." I was like,
"Okay," . . . [but] I didn't have thirty-five dollars, it wasn't like I could
just cut a check for thirty-five dollars. So, it was so funny because I
had worked at this place a year before, and they sent me a check for
pretty much thirty-five dollars. And then I was homeschooling, and it
was new to me—I was biting off more than I could chew with the
homeschooling and doing all this. And I said, "I've had a really hard
day, let's go out to eat." And I went out and spent the money. It was so
irresponsible, and we went to [a local store] to pick up some things,
and [my husband] looked behind him and told me to look at that car's
license plate. It says "Midwives!" And I said, "Wow, let's just see what

she looks like. We'll just see if I can handle this." We waited for her, and she never came out. We found an envelope, and I wrote on it "Hi, I'm looking for a midwife." [I figured,] we'll pray—if God doesn't like this, just tell him to send a wind or something and blow it off her windshield. And so she called me the next day. . . . She said, "I got your note on my car," and so I said, "Well, I'm looking for a midwife." . . . I really felt that God sent me the best midwife in Virginia. [During my birth] I kept looking up at them (laughing), I don't even know these people! I met them in a parking lot.[54]

It is significant that Paula attributed her decision to use a midwife for the first time to God—*God sent me the best midwife in Virginia*—rather than to personal choice, as many more affluent homebirthers did. Other low-income homebirthers in my study also resisted attributing their decision to hire an underground midwife solely to personal choice for fear of being pathologized and potentially punished by the state for their "bad" choices (see Chapter 5).

Implications for Activism under Neoliberalism

As governments have become less interested in protecting the social, political, and economic rights of citizens, the focus for many activists has shifted to their rights as consumers to make well-informed choices to purchase commodities and services within a free market. This has had significant implications for grassroots organizing, particularly in attempts to unite broad coalitions of socioeconomically diverse women. During my fieldwork, many participants conveyed their concerns about attempting to work together in a cross-class coalition to support midwives. For example, Jackie Grayson, one of the homebirth mothers whose story in the last chapter explained the empowerment she felt after reluctantly going to the legislature but then witnessing a positive vote on a midwifery bill, explained, "A couple people would come from more rural counties and be kind of, not really what you wanted there fighting for midwifery because they kind of perpetuated the stereotype."[55] Many middle-class and affluent advocates feared that legislators would discount their efforts to decriminalize midwives if they perceived homebirthers as rural and poor, which was historically the case in Virginia as middle-class and affluent women began to give birth in hospitals in the early to mid–twentieth century. Cindy, the wealthy "consumer advocate" who testified in the legislature "for women about childbirth," explained that, initially, she did not support midwifery, until she realized "that there was a real interest in midwifery, that it wasn't just hippies, it wasn't just total anti-establishment people, it was educated people who wanted to do the best they could for themselves and their babies."[56] As Sheryl Nestel has suggested in her study of race and midwifery in Canada, "Inclusivity may have been seen as a liability to a movement clamouring for respectability."[57] For some midwifery advocates in Virginia, this manifested itself through policing "the visible dimension of respectability" among other midwifery supporters, particularly regarding how they presented themselves within the legislature.[58]

The effect, however, was ultimately the exclusion of many low-income homebirthers from organizing efforts. Although most midwifery organizers explained that they had no intention of excluding anyone—and many earnestly shared with me their hope of convincing more women of color to join their public efforts to support midwives—divisive ideas about who should and should not be seen in the legislature in support of midwives produced deep resentment among some low-income mothers. Paula, for example, highlighted her disillusionment with the reception she received when she attended several local meetings of midwifery advocates:

> Every time that I [mentioned that] I homebirthed because I was poor . . . this one woman who always stands up [at meetings] and says, "But that's not the only reason," because they don't want to hear that within the movement. I am told not to say it's because I was poor [that I had a homebirth] because that makes you look dumb. . . . Most of the people I've seen in this movement had a lot and have had the opportunity to say they were taken care of by their parents. And I didn't come from that class. I wasn't even brought up to go to college. It wasn't an issue in my house. When I look at people in this movement, they're older, have one child, want to get the most they can out of this experience, and I think that's great, I do. Where I grew up, children were part of life, you didn't dwell about it. You were lucky to have health insurance so you could go to that doctor and do everything that looks good, you know, get [your children] all immunized on time and [make sure] they all looked nice and clean so they could get a good shot of having the teachers at school look at them. . . . The other people [in the midwifery movement] were able to travel, didn't stay in one area, have seen other ways of life, grew up in California and are in Virginia now. . . . It's definitely a social thing of having money, having time to read the books, and be able to take care of yourself. I know it's by the grace of God that I know what I do, because I did not have those opportunities.[59]

Paula describes not only the differences between herself and *the other people* supporting midwives in terms of access to reproductive choices but also *the social thing of having money,* which allowed middle-class homebirthers the *time to read books* and the resources to *have health insurance* and *take care of themselves* better than she could without *those opportunities.*

Stories such as Paula's may also explain why I never witnessed direct confrontation over socioeconomic issues or the use of the term "consumer" in public forums or organizational meetings of midwifery supporters. Many of the low-income homebirthers I interviewed said that they had just stopped coming to organizing meetings because they did not feel that their concerns were being heard. Others may have felt intimidated about mentioning financial concerns after experiencing or witnessing interactions such as the one Paula described. Middle-class organizers also frequently stated that poor women were just not part of the midwifery movement, creating perhaps a self-fulfilling prophecy. As one organizer who identified herself as a "midwifery consumer" claimed, "The issue in Virginia is a white, middle-class—white upper-middle-class even— [movement], 'cause you don't even see that many poor people. . . . We don't talk about insurance, we don't even really talk about Medicaid, we don't really talk about money being an issue."[60]

Notably, low-income women—even those who became involved in organizing efforts for midwives—remained consistent in their contention that identification as "consumers" was not a useful strategy to describe their support of midwives, particularly because it did not defend them against state intervention in their lives for making "bad (consumer) choices." As Paula explained, this has had direct implications for those who have felt "entitled" to become involved in the midwifery movement. For some low-income homebirthers, the disapproval of middle-class organizers was a significant reason not to remain involved in consumer-based advocacy. In an interview after the passage of legislation to legalize CPMs, one low-income homebirther, who had been an active supporter of midwives in the late 1990s but had since left organized groups that supported midwives, recalled:

> We were just so much more politically and socially conscious when this thing started. Then it became a consumer thing . . . that's when folks who didn't identify as consumers just left organizing groups. . . . [Now] it's about let's raise money and get influence. . . . It's not about women's rights anymore.[61]

When I asked her why she did not identify as a "consumer," she responded:

> It feels like you're going shopping and you have a right to your choices. I think of consuming as this little Pac Man going around, "oh, I'll have this' and 'I'll have that." . . . I don't want my capacity to birth to be

quantified, marketed, and packaged. . . . You know it made it this face-less thing of a purchase, instead of women making decisions about their bodies. . . . You're just trying to make midwifery one of the many "choices" and then you sanitize it to the point where it's not midwifery anymore . . . and then you call it a consumer choice.[62]

Organizers' concerns with *rais[ing] money and get[ting] influence* to make *a purchase* of midwifery care clearly did not connect with this homebirth mother's commitment to *women's rights* to make *decisions about their bodies*. Similarly, another low-income mother explained: "I'm really only a consumer when it comes to shopping—I love to shop! But when it comes to birth, the bond you have with your midwife is not about that. It's so much more."[63] Solinger has called the shift from the idea of reproductive rights to merely reproductive choices "rights lite." Indeed, choice, "a term that evoked women shoppers selecting among options in the marketplace, [was] an easier sell . . . a package less threatening or disturbing than unadulterated rights."[64]

Like the midwives discussed earlier in this chapter, organizers and middle-class homebirthers were also aware of the limitations of the term "consumer" regarding the relationship women had with their midwives, but they continued to find it politically palatable. One middle-class homebirth mother explained:

I think it [the idea of midwifery as a "consumer's right"] was useful with legislators because I think it finally puts us on equal ground of being able to talk about something that everybody could understand. . . . But I think is does take away . . . the partnership between women and their midwives.[65]

Thus identifying as consumers had the potential to put middle-class home-birthers on *equal ground* with legislators, something that most low-income homebirthers could not envision.

Although tensions between socioeconomically diverse women in organizing efforts for reproductive healthcare are hardly a new phenomenon (see Chapters 1 and 2), the neoliberal promotion of access to healthcare services as a "consumer right" has added new fuel to these existing divisions. While organizers have attempted to show legislators how midwives serve a variety of diverse communities, including those composed of poor women—at least statistically—in legislative debates, the efforts to silence discussions of poverty among grassroots organizers have left most low-income homebirthers decidedly outside of what many have described as the more "mainstream midwifery movement." Thus low-income women have found themselves in a particularly difficult position in their efforts to support midwives.

Broadly speaking, under neoliberalism individuals are expected to contribute to civil society by uncritically accepting the "consumerization" of all aspects of life.[66] Consequently, it becomes the consumer who makes change through the marketplace, not the citizen who brings about change through political engagement. Thus grassroots organizers who have attempted to convince legislators to license midwives in areas such as Virginia have found market-based arguments both strategic and politically effective. However, despite guarantees of universal rights for all citizens, the government ultimately denies access to basic rights to those who do not consume enough and are thus not deemed fully qualified as citizens.[67]

Rather than unifying activists—as was the aim of the feminists who encouraged consumer-based identification in struggles to gain reproductive rights in the 1960s and 1970s—under neoliberalism, the consumer model has highlighted the economic vulnerability of low-income women. Ultimately, the use of both *consumer* and *choice* in the context of women's healthcare speaks more broadly to whose lives and choices neoliberal policies support and whose they do not. In effect, the meaning of a right has changed under neoliberalism, and the promotion of "good" citizenship and motherhood as consumer-based identities ignores the government's role in preserving the rights of all citizens. Instead, consumers must rely on the fluctuations of other consumers' desires within the marketplace to ensure their social, political, and economic rights. Of course, as many social scientists and feminist scholars have shown, this means that those with the most financial resources receive "the best" care, whether that is perceived as access to midwives or to the most advanced new reproductive technologies, and low-income women are left without the resources to compete.

Solinger has explained the dangers of "choice" and market-based arguments for reproductive rights as they initially emerged during the activist efforts of the 1960s and 1970s:

> In theory, choice refers to an individual preference and wants to protect all women from reproductive coercion. In practice, though, choice has two faces. The contemporary language of choice promises dignity and reproductive autonomy to women with resources. For women without, the language of choice is a taunt and a threat. . . . [Thus,] "choice" has effectively blocked cross-class coalitions of women supporting each other's reproductive dignity, as Americans have come to strongly and stubbornly associate financial "independence" with legitimate choice making.[68]

Because feminist scholars were some of the first to promote consumer-based identification among midwifery advocates, it is particularly important to criti-

cally examine the challenges that emerge with the intensification of consumer rights' arguments to gain and maintain reproductive rights under neoliberalism. Yet what continues to complicate this matter considerably is that
midwives and their supporters have been successful in their efforts to legalize
and loosen restrictions on midwives in areas such as Virginia. This brings up
important questions for both scholars and activists, particularly those who
value the woman-centered care offered by midwives and the increasing interest in midwives across a broad political, religious, and socioeconomic spectrum of women. Are feminist notions of "choice" and a woman's "right to
choose" becoming diluted under neoliberalism? Do alternatives to market-
based efforts regarding reproductive healthcare reform exist?

These concerns are compounded by the recent interest among medical
institutions, insurance companies, and the government in the economic possibilities of a "new market" for midwifery services—presumably for women
with the economic ability to consume such services out of pocket or with private insurance—which has paralleled the increasing public interest in midwifery and homebirth.[69] It is important for both activists and scholars to continue to ask this question: Who will ultimately have access to this proliferation
of consumer choices? Perhaps it is time for midwifery supporters, including
the scholars who support these efforts, to refocus attention on the shared experiences of homebirthers by highlighting the respect, support, and safe care
that socioeconomically-diverse women have received from midwives. These
arguments remain powerful in both organizing efforts and legislative debates,
but the recent intensification of consumer rights strategies has largely eclipsed
these shared experiences for many low-income homebirthers. Another potentially unifying strategy that became important in Virginia during meetings of
the Governor's Work Group on Rural Obstetrical Care in 2004 involved arguments about how the low cost of midwifery care (relative to physician's and
hospital's fees for childbirth) could improve women's access to reproductive
care in "medically underserved" rural areas. In this case, midwifery supporters
from a broad range of socioeconomic backgrounds came together to highlight
the importance of midwifery in the improvement of reproductive healthcare
services.[70]

Although midwifery supporters represent a unique and proportionally
small group of reproductive healthcare advocates (since DEMs attend less
than 1 percent of all U.S. births, and CNMs attend an additional 7 percent,
mostly in the hospital),[71] the experiences within this movement hold important lessons for those who support broader struggles for women's reproductive
freedom. Not unlike the historical examples of reproductive healthcare activism that have led to uneven gains for different constituencies of women, contemporary struggles for reproductive rights under neoliberalism have the potential

to reproduce and intensify these divisions among women whose reproductive decisions are frequently distinguished not by individualized notions of "choice" but, rather, by unequal social and economic resources. Ultimately, as reproductive rights are increasingly subject to the whims of a globalizing capitalist economy, it is essential to continue to critically examine how and whether consumers' rights can intersect with efforts to secure accessible, low-cost reproductive healthcare for all women.

Epilogue
Beyond Consumer Rights

An Update on Virginia and the Future of Reproductive Freedom for All Women

Childbirth decisions should not be dictated or influenced by
what's fashionable, trendy, or the latest cause célèbre. . . .
ACOG believes that the safest place for labor, delivery, and
the immediate postpartum period is in the hospital, or
birthing center within a hospital complex . . . or [an
accredited] freestanding birthing center. . . . The main goal
should be a healthy and safe outcome for both mother and
baby. Choosing to deliver a baby at home, however, is to
place the process of giving birth over the goal of having a
healthy baby.
> —AMERICAN COLLEGE OF OBSTETRICIANS AND
> GYNECOLOGISTS, "ACOG STATEMENT ON HOME BIRTHS"

I n 2008, the American College of Obstetricians and Gynecologists (ACOG)
renewed its public relations campaign to reiterate its long-standing opposition
to homebirths. Shortly afterward, the American Medical Association (AMA)
went a step further—it endorsed ACOG's statement and vowed to develop
model legislation to potentially outlaw all homebirths in the United States.
In a smartly titled press release "Father Knows Best Meets Big Brother Is
Watching"—reminiscent of Virginia homebirth mothers' statements about their
relationships with legislators and medical officials—representatives of the Big
Push for Midwives launched a counterattack. Susan Jenkins, an attorney for
legal strategy in the Big Push for Midwives Campaign, explained:

> It's unclear what penalties the AMA will seek to impose on women
> who choose to give birth at home, either for religious, cultural, or fi-
> nancial reasons—or just because they didn't make it to the hospital in

time. What we do know, however, is that any state that enacts such a law will immediately find itself in court, since a law dictating where a woman must give birth would be a clear violation of fundamental rights to privacy and other freedoms currently protected by the U.S. Constitution.[1]

Within this tense political climate, however, organizers in states pushing for the licensure of CPMs, or seeking to revise current laws, find themselves in a difficult situation. In fact, despite Virginia CPMs' continued struggle for the legal authority to administer certain medications—RhoGAM for Rh-negative mothers, Pitocin and Methergine for postpartum hemorrhage, oxygen for emergencies, lidocaine for suturing, and vitamin K and erythromycin for newborns—they feel fortunate for their licensure law in the face of this renewed and powerful opposition to homebirth. As Brynne Potter, who played a central role in the passage of the 2005 legislation to license CPMs, wrote to a group of midwifery supporters, "Every other state that has passed legislation in the last 3 years has had major attempts to role back their law. . . . [We are] grateful that we have a law (we might not be able to pass one in the current national climate), and that we are able to practice without threat of criminal prosecution."[2]

Returning to Virginia

I returned to Virginia in 2007 to conduct follow-up interviews with midwives and their supporters to get a sense of the changes they experienced after the law licensing CPMs was passed in 2005. Midwives, as mentioned earlier, were understandably relieved to be legally recognized, though those who had been involved in the legislative push felt a continued sense of personal responsibility for making sure other midwives were happy with the law. Lingering concerns about medications weighed heavily on their minds. Midwives have also had to be vigilant about laws that have been introduced to curtail their practices, and so far they have been able to fight these laws successfully with the help of vocal "midwifery consumers." Several midwives also reported a change in the demographics of homebirthers since the passage of the law—more women with health insurance were seeking to be reimbursed for midwifery services, and some midwives had had success getting Medicaid reimbursement (though there were many hoops for both mothers and the midwives to jump through in order to do so). The CNMs were also successful in passing a law in 2006 that eliminated physician supervision as a condition for licensure, however, supervision remains a requirement for prescriptive authority, which continues to make it difficult for most CNMs to run out-of-hospital practices. Several nurse-midwives have become CPMs and are now attending homebirths. Like all CPMs, however, administering any medication now falls outside of their scope of practice under current laws. Finally, although the state legislature has offered some support for the expansion of CNM care in rural areas,[3] CNMs have also been fired from several hospitals for not being "profitable enough." Thus the situation for midwives in Virginia remains a tenuous one.

Homebirth mothers who had been involved in legislative efforts were also largely pleased—both with their legal access to midwives who attended homebirths and the sense of accomplishment they felt after successfully lobbying to change Virginia law. And women's access to midwives had also changed dramatically since 2005. Although there were no official counts of unlicensed midwives who practiced prior to the 2005 law, all the homebirthers with whom I spoke (in various areas of the state) mentioned that new midwives had begun practicing in their region. According to the Virginia Department of Health Professions, by 2010, fifty four midwives had become licensed in Virginia.[4] Several of these midwives practice in other nearby states where DEM practice is not legal (with the intent that if they are ever investigated they would be able to show that they had been legally licensed in another state, even if they were unable to be licensed in their own), but it is clear that more women have access to midwives throughout Virginia than they did prior to the 2005 legislation. Still, several of the low-income women with whom I spoke felt that not much had changed for them personally with the passage of legislation to license CPMs. Some continued to homebirth with midwives in their communities who were not CPMs (and thus unlicensed). Others worked diligently to obtain Medicaid coverage for homebirths—with mixed success.

Although groups of women in Virginia still come together in their communities to support each other in childbirth and educate others about their birth options, the majority of Virginia's grassroots organizations to support midwifery licensure have now merged into a statewide group called VABirthPAC (formerly midwivespac), a political action committee devoted to influencing, more broadly, maternal and child health policies (VABirthPAC postcard).

One particularly valuable strategy that VABirthPAC is continuing following the successful legislative effort by midwivespac to license CPMs is maintaining an electronic database of midwifery supporters—approximately 2,000 so far—organized by legislative district, which has allowed organizers to target key legislators by mobilizing constituents to contact their local representatives. One of the postcards that midwivespac distributed by mail and online to midwifery supporters across the state prior to the passage of the 2005 legislation is shown on page 143.

VABirthPAC is the political voice of concerned
Citizens who want to impact evidence-based
Maternal/Child health care policies in the
Commonwealth of Virginia.

VABirthPAC

◆   Support, propose and track legislation that impacts
    Maternal/Child health in Virginia.
◆   Raise money for organizational development and
    influence the selection, nomination, or election of any
    State office.
◆   Network with other Virginia organizations to affect change
    in Maternal/Child health.

Go to **www.vabirthpac.org** for ways you can
Contribute to **VABirthPAC** and the
Commonwealth of Virginia political process

VABirthPAC
9702 Gayton Road • PMB 261 • Richmond, VA 23233
www.vabirthpac.org

Paid for and authorized by VABirthPAC.

VABirthPAC postcard, distributed at fund-raising events.

It is also worth noting the bipartisan support that midwives and their supporters were able to generate in Virginia, which they hope to continue through
VABirthPAC. Although primary support for midwives in other states, such as
Florida, has come predominately from Democrats,[5] in Virginia the primary
patrons of bills to license CPMs have been Republicans. Many of these legislators were eager to support "pro-woman" legislation (since most did not support other reproductive rights, such as abortion or contraception). In 2004,
midwives and their supporters were particularly excited when their bill was
co-patroned (inadvertently) by Democrat Adam Ebbin, Virginia's first openly
gay legislator, and Republican Dick Black, the patron of several anti-gay and
anti-abortion bills, that same year. Organizers felt that the irony of both
legislators—who are so diametrically opposed on other issues—supporting
midwives sent a powerful message that homebirth is an issue that affects a
diverse array of women.

Dear Legislator,

Virginia is one of the few remaining states without access to the
maternity provider and setting of choice for families.

In this session you are going to have an opportunity to vote on
Legislation that would license trained home birth care providers,
Certified Professional Midwives.

Virginians want home birth and access to licensed CPMs. This need
Is evident by the increase in home births over the past decade, as well
As public testimony from the JCHC hearings in 1999, and the OB
Task Force hearings in 2004.

I support this legislation and as my representative I urge you to vote

YES for Midwives!

Signature_____ Date_____

Postcard sent to legislators by hundreds of midwifery supporters throughout Virginia
before successful legislation to license CPMs in 2005.

Pushing toward the Future

The support of homebirth and midwives is, without a doubt, an issue that
brings together women from across the political spectrum, and with a variety
of reasons—religious, cultural, personal, and financial—for choosing midwives. Within this context, the recent focus on the "consumer's right" to *hire* a
midwife—rather than women's, mothers', or citizens' rights to reproductive
healthcare access—has proved to be a palatable way to unite many of these
women. This has occurred in the United States, as I have outlined in this book,
as well as internationally. For example, the Midwifery Task Force of Ontario
(MTFO) became the Ontario Midwifery Consumer Network (OMCN) in the
1990s,[6] and a quick online search shows the proliferation of "consumer" groups
supporting midwives in Australia, New Zealand, and throughout Europe.

As discussed in the previous chapters, "consumer rights" has also become
an effective political argument in the face of hostile medical opposition in
legislative debates. However, the relationship between women's organizing for
midwifery and homebirth as "consumers" (those economically secure enough
to be able to consume midwifery services) and the contemporary political

climate surrounding reproductive rights remains a sticky one. Raymond De Vries warned nearly fifteen years ago: "For women in the upper and middle classes, these dynamics determine options available for childbirth. For women with limited resources, the midwifery-law relationship can altogether eliminate choice."[7]

So where does this leave us? Just as Virginia midwifery supporters have rightfully continued to ask throughout my research, "That's fascinating, Christa. So, what do we do *now*?" Robbie Davis-Floyd also struggled with this question as it arose in her research with national organizations of midwives striving to gain legitimacy and, for some, professionalization within the U.S. healthcare system. Her answer was deeply personal: Midwifery proponents, in their unwavering confidence that childbirth is indeed healthy and organic, inspired her to give birth to her second child at home with midwives.[8] Undeniably, I have been similarly inspired, though I also remain concerned about how we can keep this option available for the broad spectrum of women who desire midwives.

My "answer" has more to do with challenging the broader neoliberal shift away from governmental commitments to preserve all citizens' rights toward a consumer rights paradigm than it does with midwifery advocacy itself. The identification of citizens as consumers is undeniably a trend seen much more broadly than just among midwifery supporters, or even reproductive rights advocates.[9] Following the 9/11 terrorist attacks, for instance, an upsurge of "patriotic consumerism" was evident in the United States. Politicians called on Americans to "buy for one's country" and "the spectacle of such consumption emerged as a shorthand for national belonging, as proof of genuine citizenship."[10] Consumer- and market-based language was also common among politicians across the political spectrum in the debates leading up to the passage of national healthcare reform in the United States in 2010. For instance, one senator, arguing in 2009 for the "public option" to grant access to government-run insurance to "every American," suggested that, as a nation, we must "guarantee that all consumers have affordable, meaningful and accountable options available in the health insurance marketplace."[11]

Following suit, activists of many stripes have also adopted the language and strategies of consumer activism to attain maximum political impact in a government that favors this model. Instead of "go green," for instance, we now hear "buy green." Marches and rallies for issues from ending hunger to gay, lesbian, bisexual, and transgender rights now court corporate sponsors who hope to entice the new market of consumers impassioned about these issues to "shop ethically" at businesses that support (or at least are not antagonistic toward) their chosen cause. Environmental activist Raj Patel has called this "the honey trap of ethical consumerism," where one is "caught" in the belief that social change can only be achieved through consumer choices rather than through collective political action.[12]

Despite my distaste for this overall trend, I could not, in good conscience, advise those who support contemporary midwives to stop the calculated use of the term "consumer" to make their needs known to legislators who respond far more favorably to purchasing power than to appeals for the rights of women, mothers, or citizens. Yet midwifery advocates also need to remain conscious and mindful of the circumstantial alliances they make. As the history of women's activism for reproductive healthcare demonstrates, sometimes "uneasy alliances"—such as those between feminists and abolitionists in the popular health movement and conservative and progressive women in the natural childbirth movement—can be fruitful. In other cases, strategic alliances have had far more detrimental effects. Recall the alliance of early-twentieth-century feminists struggling for abortion and contraception with eugenicists who hoped these technologies would discourage women they deemed unfit (African Americans, recent immigrants, and poor women) from reproducing in order to propagate "the white race." Today, many midwifery advocates (and activists more generally) join forces with proponents of neoliberal policies in their struggle for reproductive rights, but at what cost? Will all women ultimately benefit from this partnership?

It is now more important than ever for activists and scholars of reproductive rights to revisit both the vocabulary and the ethics of advocacy strategies that can be divisive *within* organizing efforts. Notably, the participants in my study—from all socioeconomic backgrounds—began supporting midwives and homebirth because of their shared passion and commitment to natural childbirth and social change. *They have not supported midwifery merely as a pragmatic mass of consumers.* Even though my research questions all centered on political activity to support midwives, *almost every* participant in my study also related at least one life-changing story about either her own childbirth experience or attending a midwife-assisted homebirth. Whether a moving account of birth with a midwife in the home, a frightening but protected transfer from the home to the hospital with a midwife, a positive experience in the hospital with a supportive physician or nurse-midwife, or a terrifying hospital birth, most participants said they began to support midwifery because of these experiences. Clearly, for these women, motherhood is not merely a consumer status. Many saw their stories and shared experiences through childbirth as the basis for their political power. And most women described not only their own passion for homebirth and midwives but their heartfelt aspiration to make midwives and homebirth available to *all* women.

As Sheryl Ruzek reminds us, however, "Ideologies of inclusiveness and commitments to extending health and medical care benefits to all women across class and race lines are credible only if they are conceivably attainable."[13] One primary drawback of a "consumer rights" strategy for access to homebirth midwifery is that gaining this access as "consumers" has the potential to limit these services to only those who are ultimately able to afford them. Consequently, the adoption of "consumer rights" as an advocacy strategy was compelling and effective only for some midwifery supporters in my study, primarily those who were more affluent. In an effort dedicated to bringing what the Midwives Alliance of North America describes as "access to midwifery care to all women,"[14] however, this is not a sustainable strategy. As previous struggles to expand the focus of reproductive rights to include the concerns of women of color have shown us,

> there is a tendency among feminists, both contemporary and historical, to suggest that by defending the rights of white, middle-class women to bodily integrity and sovereignty, women of color and poor women's rights will also be defended. . . . Feminists fail in their ultimate goal—to ensure the rights of *all* women—if they do not make a first priority the needs of those who have the least access to reproductive freedom.[15]

In light of the troubling legacy of women's struggles for reproductive options throughout the past century, which led to uneven successes for women whose access to reproductive services was already stratified by race and class, we cannot afford to repeat this history by claiming to be "sisters in struggle" and at the same time employing divisive organizing strategies. Frankly, I have higher hopes for those who support the extent to which midwives have gone—both historically and presently—to make their services available to all women who seek their care. Even though "consumer" identity and consumption-based metaphors may be useful politically with legislators and medical officials, they no longer need to be central to the descriptions of our grassroots organizations and the local, national, and international events to support midwives.

Yet it is not enough to just point out the limits of neoliberalism and consumer rights rhetoric and to merely substitute other terms or slogans. Nor is it enough to "shop ethically"—either by hiring midwives or buying goods from companies or individuals one supports. Of course, being conscious of one's individual consumption is clearly important, but there are larger issues that need attention within the broader movement for reproductive rights. Today's reproductive rights activists—including those who support access to midwives—must ground themselves in a historical perspective on women's activism for reproductive healthcare that acknowledges the exclusions and tensions that have impacted previous struggles. As demonstrated in this book, the racial and class inequities that have existed historically have *intensified* under neoliberalism—they are not inherently new.

Thus it is not only the recent political and economic developments that have privileged "consumer rights" that must be challenged but also the long-standing race- and class-based exclusion that has divided, and frequently continues to divide, reproductive healthcare activists. As women of color who are active in reproductive rights struggles have powerfully argued,[16] and as I have echoed in this book, the fight for women's access to reproductive rights, including midwifery, must be waged within the context of a broader social and reproductive justice perspective. It is through a commitment to justice—not merely individualized claims to consumer rights—that access to midwives and other reproductive options will become a reality for *all* women. In fact, it is precisely this individual rights discourse that can blind us to injustices and exclusions.

Our goal of attaining reproductive freedom is not completed if we stop merely at the protection of individuals and their choices. If we do so then we miss entire categories of people, those who do not have the same access to resources and choices as most middle-class and affluent women do. Although a "consumer rights" approach may be effective in a neoliberal environment, reproductive rights activists must be vigilant about making sure their organizing efforts include a broad range of reproductive experiences and levels of access. For those who believe in reproductive justice for all women, motherhood and pregnancy cannot be reduced to a consumer status.[17] It is my hope that as the effort to support midwives continues throughout the nation and beyond, we also continue to be attentive to this uneven history and to refine our strategies. A push for midwives that is grounded in a sincere commitment to enhancing reproductive justice for all women has the potential to enhance reproductive rights for a much broader spectrum of women—*including* their ability to access the exceptional and empowering care that midwives provide.

Notes

NOTES ON RESEARCH AND ACTIVISM

1. Several feminist ethnographers were particularly influential to me as I undertook this challenging task; see Abu-Lughod, *Veiled Sentiments;* Fraser, *African American Midwifery in the South;* Layne, *Motherhood Lost;* Davis, *Battered Black Women and Welfare Reform;* Gray, *Out in the Country.*

2. Haraway, "Situated Knowledges."

3. Declerq, Paine, and Winter, "Home Birth in the United States, 1989–1992, 480.

4. Beginning as an undergraduate, I was inspired by feminist authors' personal interrogation of their particular subject positions in relation to the broader feminist movement. See, for instance: Lorde, *Zami;* Anzaldúa, *Borderlands/La Frontera;* and the authors in Behar and Gordon, *Women Writing Culture.*

5. Nestel, *Obstructed Labour,* 5, emphasis in original.

6. Abu-Lughod, "Writing against Culture," 141, emphasis in original.

7. "Femme" is a term commonly used in U.S. lesbian communities to refer to women who dress and behave in ways regarded as traditionally feminine or effeminate. For a more nuanced discussion and a social history of this term, see Nestle, *A Restricted Country.*

8. This participant subsequently invited me to stay with her family on several occasions and also shared with me the experience of a local midwife who had had a relationship with a woman. While this midwife was involved in a long-term relationship with a man when I met her, when she was "outed" regarding her earlier relationship with a woman to some of her more conservative clients, many of these clients decided to end their personal and professional relationships with her. My friend, deeply saddened by this, felt that other homebirthers' betrayal of her midwife was unprincipled, and equally inappropriate in her friendship with me.

INTRODUCTION: PUSHING FOR MIDWIVES

1. "Direct-entry midwife" (DEM) is a term that originated in Europe to refer to midwives who entered directly into their profession, often through apprenticeship, as opposed to those who became midwives through nursing schools. The category includes licensed midwives (LMs) in states where midwifery is legal and regulated, certified professional midwives and certified midwives (CPMs and CMs, respectively, two national certifications for DEMs), and those who label themselves traditional midwives, empirical midwives, community-based midwives, and domiciliary midwives (though the "domiciliary midwives" could also refer to nurse-midwives who attend births in a home setting). The terms "lay midwife" and "untrained midwife" are also widely used by medical and government officials, though most contemporary midwives find these terms offensive. Though the term "DEM" represents a variety of birthcare practitioners trained and certified in different ways, it is widely understood by grassroots organizers as a coherent group of midwives who specialize in attending homebirths.

2. Big Push for Midwives, "Number Two with a Bullet," press release, September 1, 2008.

3. Collaborating groups include the National Association of Certified Professional Midwives (NACPM), Midwives Alliance of North America (MANA), Citizens for Midwifery (CfM), the International Center for Traditional Childbearing (ICTC), North American Registry of Midwives (NARM), and the Midwifery Education Accreditation Council (MEAC); MAMA Campaign, "The Midwives and Mothers in Action (MAMA) Campaign Is Launched!"

4. MacDonald, "Tradition as a Political Symbol," 60.

5. Fiedler and Davis-Floyd, "Midwifery as a Reproductive Right," 136. See also Block, *Pushed!* which explicitly describes "birthing rights" as reproductive rights. Specific to midwives, she writes, "Many of the illegal home-birth midwives, even those who are vehemently opposed to abortion, defend their criminal activity in terms of protecting women's *choices*" (268, emphasis in original).

6. For the most up-to-date information, see the Big Push for Midwives, "The Push States," available at www.thebigpushformidwives.org/index.cfm/fuseaction/home.state Status/index.htm.

7. Nurse-midwives, who are trained first as nurses and then receive advanced training in nurse-midwifery, began practicing in the United States in the 1920s and 1930s—primarily to offer birthcare to women in impoverished communities. For example, the Frontier Nursing School, established by Mary Breckinridge, was vital to the improvement of maternal and infant mortality rates among poor women in Appalachia; for more information, see Rooks, *Midwifery and Childbirth in America*, 37. During the mid-1900s, the rise in homecare by nurse-midwives contributed to the decline of community-based midwives in many areas, and public health officials' efforts to replace "lay midwives" with nurse-midwives were successful in many areas by the 1970s (in Virginia, such legislation was passed in 1976). For additional exploration of this history, see Susie, *In the Way of Our Grandmothers*, 72; Mathews, "Killing the Medical Self-Help Tradition," 74; and Fraser, *African American Midwifery in the South*, 39. The most recent data from the National Center for Health Statistics

(2006) indicates that CNMs practice primarily in the hospital, attending approximately 7 percent of births in the United States; see Martin et al., "Births," 16.

8. Virginia Chapter of the American College of Nurse Midwives, "About the VA Chapter."

9. In fact, Katherine Prown, campaign manager for the Big Push for Midwives, was originally an active supporter of midwives in Virginia during the early stages of organizing, and Brynne Potter, who was a central public figure in Virginia's legislative struggle for midwives, now sits on the board of directors for the North American Registry of Midwives (NARM) since receiving her CPM credential in 2005.

10. Midwives Alliance of North America, "MANA Position Statements."

11. Ginsburg and Rapp, *Conceiving the New World Order*; see also Colen, "'With Respect and Feelings'."

12. Klassen, *Blessed Events,* 251, emphasis added.

13. Solinger, *Pregnancy and Power,* 139; see also Solinger, *Beggars and Choosers.*

14. Solinger, *Pregnancy and Power,* 138.

15. Solinger, *Beggars and Choosers,* 6.

16. Cross, *An All-Consuming Century,* 157–158.

17. Asian Communities for Reproductive Justice, "A New Vision for Advancing Our Movement." See also, Nelson, *Women of Color and the Reproductive Rights Movement*; Silliman et al., *Undivided Rights*; Smith, "Beyond Pro-Choice versus Pro-Life"; Solinger, *Pregnancy and Power.*

18. Smith, "Beyond Pro-Choice versus Pro-Life," 129.

19. Rothman, "Caught in the Current," 283.

20. Taylor, Layne, and Wozniak, *Consuming Motherhood.*

21. Rothman, "Caught in the Current," 279.

22. Davis-Floyd, "Ups, Downs, and Interlinkages," 23.

23. Davis-Floyd, "Consuming Childbirth," 214.

24. MacDonald, "Postmodern Negotiations with Medical Technology," 261.

25. See, for example, Bourgeault, *Push!,* xii.

26. Klassen, "Mothers between God and Mammon," 250.

27. Harvey, *A Brief History of Neoliberalism,* 42.

28. See, for example, Ehrenreich and English, *For Her Own Good*; Ruzek, *The Women's Health Movement*; Morgen, *Into Our Own Hands.*

29. Weisman, *Women's Health Care.*

30. Fraser, "Modern Bodies, Modern Minds," 55; see also Cobb, "Incorporation and Change"; Susie, *In the Way of Our Grandmothers*; Mathews, "Killing the Medical Self-Help Tradition among African Americans."

31. See, for example, Arms, *Immaculate Deception*; Litoff, *American Midwives*; Rothman, *In Labor*; and the recently updated and revised version by Simonds, Rothman, and Norman, *Laboring On*; Sullivan and Weitz, *Labor Pains*; Cassidy, *Birth.*

32. Fraser, "Modern Bodies, Modern Minds," 55.

33. Canadian historians and social scientists have also been at the forefront of efforts to reconstruct the history of midwifery with broader attention to the diversity of women's and midwives' experiences in Canada. See, for example, Biggs, "Rethinking the History of Midwifery in Canada," 17; Nestel, *Obstructed Labour.*

34. Morgen, *Into Our Own Hands,* 68.

35. Nelson, *Women of Color and the Reproductive Rights Movement*; Silliman et al., *Undivided Rights*.

36. This is in sharp contrast to the ways that neoliberalism has become part of the vernacular in other areas of the world, such as Latin America and Korea. In the U.S., neoliberalism is frequently understood as a part of longstanding American ideals, such as freedom and individuality, and thus it has not become part of our common political language. My thanks to Martin Manalansan for highlighting this important difference.

37. See, for example, Harvey, *A Brief History of Neoliberalism*.

38. For instance, neoliberal policies aimed at liberalizing both national economies and the global financial market were first embraced and implemented by some of the most politically conservative forces in the world during the 1980s (Ronald Reagan in the United States, Margaret Thatcher in England, and Deng Xaioping in China) and opposed by political liberals throughout the world (for additional discussion, see Harvey, *A Brief History of Neoliberalism*). Yet it was Democratic president Bill Clinton who implemented neoliberal efforts to privatize welfare in the 1990s, such as the Personal Responsibility and Work Opportunity Reconciliation Act (PRWORA), ending Aid to Families with Dependent Children (AFDC), which had provided the primary economic safety net for poor women and their children since 1935. For a rich ethnographic portrait of the effects PRWORA has had on women trying to leave abusive relationships, see Davis, *Battered Black Women and Welfare Reform*.

39. Gill, *Teetering on the Rim*, 3.

40. Two useful ethnographic examples documenting these effects are Maskovsky, "'Managing' the Poor," and Lyon-Callo, *Inequality, Poverty, and Neoliberal Governance*.

41. Goode and Maskovsky, *The New Poverty Studies*, 6.

42. Roth, "Justice Denied." This dramatic increase is often attributed to "mandatory sentencing" laws, which require minimum sentences for particular crimes, such as the possession of small amounts of illegal drugs (without intent to sell) or association with men who are convicted on drug charges.

43. Harvey, *A Brief History of Neoliberalism*, 3.

44. Foucault, *Discipline and Punish*.

45. Kingfisher and Maskovsky, "Introduction."

46. Ibid., 120.

47. Grewal, *Transnational America*.

48. Nestel, *Obstructed Labour*, 70.

49. The Big Push for Midwives, "The Push States." In the remaining twenty-three states, the District of Columbia and Puerto Rico, midwives can be subject to criminal prosecution for practicing medicine, nursing, or midwifery without a license. See Davis-Floyd and Johnson, *Mainstreaming Midwifery* for a more thorough analysis of the status of DEMs in selected states.

50. Klassen, *Blessed Events*.

51. Biggs, "Rethinking the History of Midwifery in Canada," 19.

52. Hoebel and Weaver, *Anthropology and the Human Experience*, 12–13.

53. Clifford and Marcus, *Writing Culture*, 3.

54. Stacey, "Can There Be a Feminist Ethnography?" 22; see also Visweswaran, *Fictions of Feminist Ethnography*, and "Histories of Feminist Ethnography."

55. Abu-Lughod, "Can There Be a Feminist Ethnography?"

56. See, for example, Anzaldúa, *Borderlands/La Frontera*; Harrison, *Decolonizing Anthropology*; Mullings, *On Our Own Terms*; Gordon, "Worlds of Consequences"; Mohanty, *Feminism without Borders*.

57. Harrison, "Feminist Methodology," 25.

58. Sanford and Angel-Ajani, *Engaged Observer*; Holland et al., *Local Democracy under Siege*; Hale, *Engaging Contradictions*.

59. Sanford, "Introduction" to *Engaged Observer,* 14.

60. Dána-Ain Davis notes, "My association with anthropologists and activists has revealed that some anthropologists may use their research as a stepping stone to direct engagement with activism. But just as commonly, I have found that many activists become anthropologists"; see "Knowledge in the Service of a Vision," 236.

61. Gordon, "Worlds of Consequences"; Baker, *From Savage to Negro*.

62. Waterston and Vesperi, *Anthropology off the Shelf.*

63. Davis, "Knowledge in the Service of a Vision."

64. Hale, *Engaging Contradictions,* 4.

65. See also Lassiter, *The Chicago Guide to Collaborative Ethnography.*

66. I recorded and transcribed these events for my own linguistic analysis and also to provide transcripts to organizers, who utilized them in successive years to craft responses to common arguments against pro-midwifery legislation.

67. I take this cue in part from historian Rickie Solinger, who notes in her history of reproductive politics in the United States, *Pregnancy and Power*, that knowing about history (whether distant or relatively recent, in the case of my ethnographic work) "is a collective project that depends on the work of many people" (25). In addition to acknowledging how participants in my research have contributed to this project, I also recognize the scholars who have done so.

68. George Marcus describes multi-sited ethnography, or what he calls mobile ethnography, as an effort to explore "an object of study that cannot be accounted for ethnographically by remaining focused on a single site of intensive investigation. It develops instead a strategy or design of research that acknowledges macrotheoretical concepts and narratives of the world system but does not rely on them for the contextual architecture framing a set of subjects"; see "Ethnography in/of the World System," 96.

69. Commonwealth of Virginia, Department of Health, Center for Health Statistics, "Resident Live Home Births by Zip Code."

70. Although these interviews focused primarily on mothers who had had at least one homebirth, I also interviewed political lobbyists and several fathers, grandfathers, and grandmothers who had witnessed the homebirths of loved ones and subsequently became supporters of midwives. All but two participants had children who were born at home or had used a midwife in another setting.

71. Midwifery supporters were understandably cautious about protecting their midwives, as well as their own integrity, and many indicated that they had had negative experiences with reporters and/or past researchers. In addition, during my fieldwork, a heated discussion developed about privacy on a national midwifery Listserv—after a researcher in another state quoted e-mail posts as "public documents" without consulting their authors. Midwives and their supporters on the list were justifiably concerned about their safety and privacy; many felt that the researcher had overstepped her bounds by exploiting the openness of the midwifery community for her own academic ends. The author respectfully defended her choice—the Listserv was public at the

time of the original posts (and later became private), and the e-mail authors' full names and addresses did not appear on the posts, which made contact for informed consent difficult, if not impossible. Nevertheless, this deliberation prompted my own meticulous searches for permission when quoting Listserv correspondence.

72. Geertz, "Thick Description."

73. Participants in my study reported political affiliations that were equally split between "liberal" and "conservative," aligning with a variety of political parties, including Republicans, Democrats, Greens, and Libertarians. They stated religious affiliations such as agnostic, atheist, Buddhist, Christian (Assembly of God, Catholic, Episcopalian, Lutheran, "New Age" Christian, Presbyterian, Protestant, Quaker, Reform Christian, Southern Baptist, and Unitarian Universalist), "Goddess Religion," Jewish, Native American spirituality, pagan, and Taoist. See Klassen, *Blessed Events*, for more information on the political and religious diversity of contemporary homebirthers in North America.

74. I use the terms "rural" and "urban," as they seem most descriptively relevant to the areas where participants in my study lived during my fieldwork, although not in any formal sense.

75. Declerq, Paine, and Winter, "Home Birth in the United States," 480.

76. Schor, *The Overspent American*; Bobel, *The Paradox of Natural Mothering*.

77. Based on the U.S. Census Bureau, "Income and Poverty in 1999."

78. Based on the U.S. Census Bureau, "Poverty Thresholds in 1999."

79. Three participants had Ph.D.s, five had master's degrees (four of these were CNMs), eight had completed some graduate work, two had B.S. degrees, five had B.A. degrees, eleven had attended some college, two had high school diplomas, one had a GED, and two had completed a few years of high school.

80. Of the midwives in my study, one CNM was practicing in a hospital during my research, two CNMs practiced in birth centers and clients' homes, and three were underground DEMs who attended only homebirths. Three others were student midwives (one was in school to become a CNM, and two were apprenticing with local DEMs), five were licensed as CNMs but could not secure jobs offering birthcare services, and two had previously practiced as DEMs but had quit because of the current political and legal climate in Virginia.

81. U.S. Census Bureau, "Income and Poverty in 1999."

82. Mullings, "Households Headed by Women"; Amott and Matthaei, *Race, Gender, and Work*; Naples, *Grassroots Warriors*; Farmer, *Infections and Inequalities*; Mwaria, "Diversity in the Context of Health and Illness"; Susser, "Poverty and Homelessness in U.S. Cities"; Davis, *Battered Black Women and Welfare Reform*.

83. My use of terms such as "low-income," "middle-class," and "affluent" to describe midwifery supporters is intended to be descriptive of these broader experiences.

84. Davis-Floyd, Pigg, and Cosminsky, "Daughters of Time," 106.

CHAPTER 1: HISTORIES OF STRUGGLE

1. Ginsburg and Rapp, *Conceiving the New World Order*.

2. See Martin, *The Woman in the Body*; Sawicki, *Disciplining Foucault*, esp. chap. 4, "Disciplining Mothers: Feminism and the New Reproductive Technologies"; Lock and Kaufert, *Pragmatic Women and Body Politics*.

3. See Foucault, *The History of Sexuality, Volume 1,* 95–96.

4. See, for example, Jolly and Ram, *Borders of Being;* Inhorn and Van Balen, *Infertility around the Globe.*

5. Davis-Floyd, *Birth as an American Rite of Passage,* 47.

6. See, for example: Arms, *Immaculate Deception;* Litoff, *American Midwives;* Rothman, *In Labor* and the recently updated and revised version by Simonds, Rothman, and Norman, *Laboring On;* Sullivan and Weitz, *Labor Pains;* Cassidy, *Birth.*

7. Biggs, "Rethinking the History of Midwifery in Canada," 17.

8. Weisman, *Women's Health Care,* 38.

9. For additional discussion, see Shryock, *Medicine in America,* 111–125; Ehrenreich and English, *For Her Own Good,* 48; Baer, *Biomedicine and Alternative Healing Systems in America,* 14–21.

10. Edwards and Waldorf, *Reclaiming Birth,* 151.

11. Haller, *Medical Protestants,* 47–48; Baer, *Biomedicine and Alternative Healing,* 14.

12. Baxandall, Gordon, and Reverby, *America's Working Women,* 39.

13. Ehrenreich and English, *For Her Own Good,* 56.

14. Haller, *Medical Protestants,* 47–48; Baer, *Biomedicine and Alternative Healing,* 14.

15. For further information, see Ehrenreich and English, *For Her Own Good,* 59; Baer, *Biomedicine and Alternative Healing,* 12.

16. Rothstein, *American Physicians in the Nineteenth Century,* 160; Numbers, "Do-It-Yourself the Sectarian Way," 90.

17. Ehrenreich and English, *For Her Own Good,* 49.

18. Baxandall, Gordon, and Reverby, *America's Working Women,* 39.

19. Edwards and Waldorf, *Reclaiming Birth,* 151.

20. Baer, *Biomedicine and Alternative Healing,* 36–37.

21. Ehrenreich and English, *For Her Own Good,* 88; Mullings, "Inequality and African American Health Status," 156.

22. Baer, *Biomedicine and Alternative Healing,* 36.

23. Ehrenreich and English, *For Her Own Good,* 61–62.

24. Ibid., 185; Wertz and Wertz, *Lying-In,* 202.

25. See Ginsburg, *Contested Lives,* 23. During the eighteenth and nineteenth centuries, physicians, herbalists, midwives, and even dentists and veterinarians prescribed various herbal preparations to induce abortion or to serve as contraception; see Riddle, *Contraception and Abortion from the Ancient World to the Renaissance,* 163. These included emmenagogues (to bring on the menstrual flow) and implantation preventers such as ergot, rue, Queen Anne's lace, oil of tansy, oil of savin (juniper), pennyroyal, artemisia (wormwood), and blue cohosh. Additionally, some practitioners attempted to induce abortion manually, either by inserting instruments (such as syringes) into the vagina or through the external manipulation of the pregnant woman's abdomen. For additional information, see also McGregor, *Herbal Birth Control,* and Solinger, *Pregnancy and Power,* 121.

26. Gordon, *Woman's Body, Woman's Right,* 54; Ginsburg, *Contested Lives,* 24.

27. Mohr, *Abortion in America,* 86; Ginsburg, *Contested Lives,* 24.

28. Edwin M. Hale, a physician who wrote extensively on the "homeopathic treatment of abortion" in the mid-1800s, first suggested that one in five pregnancies ended

in abortion and later shifted this estimate upward; see Mohr, *Abortion in America,* 76–79. Notably, the widespread use of abortion in the 1800s precipitated a very different social and political response than the later upsurge in the use of abortion during the late twentieth century. As Ginsburg explained in *Contested Lives,* 27: "Whereas in the 1970s evidence of women's widespread use of abortion was used to *justify* efforts to demand its legalization, in the nineteenth century the same trend became a call for criminalizing the practice."

29. Solinger, *Pregnancy and Power,* 69.

30. Mohr, *Abortion in America,* 147; Luker, *Abortion and the Politics of Motherhood,* 31.

31. Borst, *Catching Babies,* 154. Notably, midwives convicted of providing abortions were dealt with far more harshly than doctors. Borst's research in Wisconsin showed that the State Medical Practice Board permanently revoked the registration of midwives for performing an "illegal operation," although seven of the eleven physicians' licenses that were revoked for similar crimes were reinstated, "including those of two of the four doctors who served prison sentences for manslaughter" (ibid., 155).

32. Weisman, *Women's Health Care,* 56.

33. Petchesky, *Abortion and Woman's Choice,* 81.

34. Weisman, *Women's Health Care,* 55.

35. Ginsburg, *Contested Lives,* 29.

36. Ibid.

37. Mohr, *Abortion in America,* 110–111; see also Gordon, "Voluntary Motherhood."

38. Gordon, "Voluntary Motherhood," 105.

39. Ginsburg, *Contested Lives,* 29; Ehrenreich and English, *For Her Own Good,* 320.

40. Ross, "African-American Women and Abortion," 148.

41. Matthews, *The Rise of the New Woman,* 122.

42. See Petchesky, *Abortion and Woman's Choice,* 83–90.

43. Solinger, *Pregnancy and Power,* 141–142.

44. Weisman, *Women's Health Care,* 56.

45. Petchesky, *Abortion and Woman's Choice,* 73. Later, as Nazi eugenic policies gained support in Germany during the 1930s, Nancy Ordover explains in *American Eugenics: Race, Queer Anatomy, and the Science of Nationalism* (41) that many U.S. eugenicists "proudly anointed their own efforts as the predecessor for what was unfolding in Germany." In fact, it was an American, Harry Laughlin, who proposed the national registry of aliens and compulsory sterilization for "unfit" mothers, that served as "the partial blueprint for Germany's Hereditary Health Law [1933], under which two million people were sterilized during the twelve years of the Third Reich" (ibid., 30). Ordover also notes that the overt, race-based eugenics in Nazi Germany no doubt gave some U.S. eugenicists pause; however, others used Nazi eugenics as a yardstick to justify U.S. proposals for class-, race-, and disability-based sterilization as tamer—and therefore more tolerable—in comparison (ibid., 160).

46. Gordon, *Woman's Body, Woman's Right*; Ross, "African-American Women and Abortion"; Solinger, *Pregnancy and Power.*

47. Robinson, *Seventy Birth Control Clinics,* 44.

48. Ibid., as cited in Gordon, *Woman's Body, Woman's Right,* 286–287.

49. Ross, "African-American Women and Abortion," 147.

50. See also Petchesky, *Abortion and Woman's Choice*, 130.

51. Ross, "African-American Women and Abortion," 150.

52. Gordon, *Woman's Body, Woman's Right*, 354; Nelson, *Women of Color and the Reproductive Rights Movement*; Silliman et al., *Undivided Rights*, 8–9.

53. Chemical anesthesia was first introduced into American obstetric practice in 1847. Initially, white women rejected the use of ether and chloroform, largely because of the prevailing belief that pain in childbirth was natural. As childbirth became more medicalized, however, women's attitudes began to change. Physicians explained that women, particularly affluent women, had become less able to withstand pain and that pain medication would allow childbirth—as Margarete Sandelowski has explained in *Pain, Pleasure, and American Childbirth* (9)—"to be natural again."

54. Ibid., 11.

55. Litoff, *American Midwives*, 69; Wertz and Wertz, *Lying-In*, 150.

56. Sandelowski, *Pain, Pleasure, and American Childbirth*, 13.

57. Ibid., 28.

58. Leavitt, *Brought to Bed*, 131.

59. Borst, *Catching Babies*, 57.

60. Rooks, *Midwifery and Childbirth in America*, 17.

61. Langston, "Diagnosis and Normal Delivery," 381.

62. Fraser, *African American Midwifery in the South*, 95–96.

63. Stillman, "Painless Childbirth," 15.

64. Schmalhauser, "The Twilight Sleep for Women," 234–235.

65. Wertz and Wertz, *Lying-In*, 152.

66. Ibid.

67. Leupp and Hendrick, "Twilight Sleep in America," 172–173. As the advent of twilight sleep contributed to the decline in homebirths for women who could afford access to it during the early twentieth century, it also contributed to the displacement of midwives who were regarded as unqualified to perform the technique; see Leavitt, *Brought to Bed*, 135; Rooks, *Midwifery and Childbirth in America*, 22. Once twilight sleep was well established as an advantage of hospital birthing, activists associated with the natural childbirth movement exposed the dangers of neonatal depression that resulted from the use of twilight sleep, ending its dispensation in the 1960s; see Wertz and Wertz's *Lying-In*, 181. Inhaled anesthetics had largely replaced twilight sleep by this time, and during the latter part of the twentieth century, the intravenous injection of analgesics (general pain relievers, under which the patient remained conscious), the epidural administration of local anesthetics, and the use of pudendal and paracervical blocks (which numb only the area around the perineum) became more commonplace.

68. Ladd-Taylor, "'Grannies' and 'Spinsters'" 258.

69. Fraser, *African American Midwifery in the South*, 258; see also Mullings, "Inequality and African American Health Status."

70. Weisman, *Women's Health Care*, 60.

71. Wertz and Wertz, *Lying-In*, 209.

72. Shryock, *Medicine in America*, 117.

73. Skocpol, *Protecting Soldiers and Mothers*, 481.

74. Sullivan and Weitz, *Labor Pains*, 13.

75. Chafe, *The American Woman,* 28.

76. Wertz and Wertz, *Lying-In,* 209.

77. Ibid.

78. Fraser, *African American Midwifery in the South,* 52.

79. Tom, "The Evolution of Nurse-Midwifery," 7.

80. Parsons, "Child Hygiene and Public Health Nursing," 285.

81. Parnall, "Nursing and the Health of the Future," 576.

82. Solinger, *Pregnancy and Power,* 92.

83. Irving (1942), *Safe Deliverance,* 140-167, as cited in Wertz and Wertz, *Lying-In,* 133.

84. Leavitt, *Brought to Bed,* 269.

85. De Vries, *Making Midwives Legal,* 50.

86. Mongeau, "The 'Granny' Midwife," 497.

87. Leavitt, *Brought to Bed,* 297.

88. Lee, *Granny Midwives and Black Women Writers,* 42.

89. Lombardo, "Eugenic Sterilization in Virginia"; Ordover, *American Eugenics,* xxvi–xxvii; Solinger, *Pregnancy and Power,* 90.

90. Ross, "African-American Women and Abortion," 150.

91. Ladd-Taylor, "'Grannies' and 'Spinsters,'" 260; Rooks, *Midwifery and Childbirth in America,* 26.

92. Wertz and Wertz, *Lying-In,* 212; see also Dougherty, "Southern Midwifery and Organized Health Care," 115.

93. Ladd-Taylor, "'Grannies' and 'Spinsters.'" 262.

94. Many contemporary African Americans avoid the use of the term "granny." Fraser has explained in *African American Midwifery in the South* (11) that many associate granny "with such terms as 'Uncle' or 'Aunt,' which white southerners used to avoid addressing older African Americans as 'Mr.' or 'Mrs.'" Physicians also used the term to devalue African American midwives. Wertz and Wertz quote one example in *Lying-In* (216) of a doctor's campaign during the early 1900s that involved the distribution of pamphlets featuring dark photographs of alleged midwives, captioned "A 'granny' of the far South. Ignorant and superstitious, a survival of the 'magic doctors' of the West Coast of Africa." Similarly, many middle-class women joined the campaign against "granny midwifery" by making use of their affiliations with newspapers and magazines. For example, Carolyn Conant van Blarcom reviled granny midwifery in her article "Rat Pie among the Black Midwives of the South."

95. Brown and Toussaint, *Mama's Little Baby,* 99. Notably, African American women did not see all midwives in their communities in such a positive light. Gertrude Fraser explains in *African American Midwifery in the South* (141) that women distinguished between "good" and "bad" midwives as they recollected stories about childbirth in their communities during the early 1900s. Indeed, some midwives inspired a good deal of fear in their communities because of their spiritual connections and their conjurer abilities (ibid., 144).

96. Sullivan and Weitz, *Labor Pains,* 13.

97. Dougherty, "Southern Midwifery," 116–118.

98. Fraser, *African American Midwifery in the South,* 35.

99. Mathews, "Killing the Medical Self-Help Tradition among African Americans," 67.

100. Ladd-Taylor, "'Grannies' and 'Spinsters,'" 259.

101. Fraser, *African American Midwifery in the South,* 235–236; see also Martin, *The Woman in the Body,* 186.

102. Ladd-Taylor, "'Grannies' and 'Spinsters,'" 266.

103. Smith and Holmes, *Listen to Me Good,* 35.

104. Fraser, *African American Midwifery in the South,* 129.

105. Wertz and Wertz, *Lying-In,* 210; see also Taylor, "Social Movement Continuity," who argues that once suffrage was achieved, emerging ideological differences in the women's movement "divided militant from moderate suffragists and those who saw winning the vote as a means from those who saw it as an end" (763).

106. Litoff, *American Midwives,* 100; see also Lemons, *The Woman Citizen,* 172–176; Matthews, *The Rise of the New Woman,* 163.

107. Edwards and Waldorf, *Reclaiming Birth,* 155.

108. See, for example, Morgen, "'It's the Whole Power of the City against Us!'"; Morgen, *Into Our Own Hands;* Silliman et al., *Undivided Rights.*

109. Schoen, "Reconceiving Abortion," 349. See also Kaplan, *The Story of Jane,* which describes the Jane Collective, a group that provided underground abortion services in the 1960s and early 1970s and Ginsburg, *Contested Lives,* which documents her ethnographic research with both pro-life and pro-choice activists in Fargo, North Dakota, during the 1980s. These works provide an important contrast to characterizations of a more unified women's health "mega-movement," such as Weisman describes in *Women's Health Care.*

CHAPTER 2: THE BIRTH OF CONSUMER ACTIVISM FOR MIDWIVES

1. See Bourgeault, Benoit, and Davis-Floyd, *Reconceiving Midwifery,* especially Biggs's chapter "Rethinking the History of Midwifery in Canada" and Nestel's chapter "The Boundaries of Professional Belonging." Regarding reproductive politics more broadly, see Solinger, *Pregnancy and Power.*

2. Biggs, "Rethinking the History," 17–18. Biggs's initial history was published in 1983 as Catherine L. Biggs, "The Case of the Missing Midwives," and reprinted in 1990 in *Delivering Motherhood.* In her later work in 2004, Biggs "retells" this history to include the experiences not only of English midwives in Canada but also of midwives who came from aboriginal communities and immigrated to Canada from other European countries. Sociologist Sheryl Nestel, in "The Boundaries of Professional Belonging," further addresses "the limits of global sisterhood" among contemporary Canadian midwives through her work with midwives who have recently immigrated to Canada from Asia, Africa, Latin America, and the Caribbean (296). See also Nestel, *Obstructed Labour.*

3. Joan Mathews and Kathleen Zadak describe the alternative birth movement as "a consumer reaction to paternalistic and mechanistic medical obstetrical practices," and they note in "The Alternative Birth Movement in the United States" that "consumer dissatisfaction" emerged initially in the 1940s (39, 42).

4. Solinger, *Pregnancy and Power,* 12.

5. Sandelowski, *Pain, Pleasure, and American Childbirth,* 55.

6. Leavitt, "'Science' Enters the Birthing Room," 297.

7. Dick-Read, *Childbirth without Fear* and *No Time for Fear;* Lamaze, *Painless Childbirth.*

8. Kitzinger, *The Experience of Childbirth,* 19.

9. Ibid.; Kahn, *Bearing Meaning,* 310.

10. Karmel, *Thank You, Dr. Lamaze.*

11. Kahn, *Bearing Meaning,* 310; see also Mead, *Blackberry Winter,* 295.

12. Klassen, *Blessed Events,* 29.

13. Cassidy, *Birth,* 154.

14. Edwards and Waldorf, *Reclaiming Birth,* 48.

15. Nestel, "'Other Mothers,'" 8.

16. Kahn, *Bearing Meaning,* 312; see also Edwards and Waldorf, *Reclaiming Birth,* 48.

17. Margaret Mead, in her autobiography *Blackberry Winter* (300), describes her own attempt to recreate a "natural" childbirth experience in a U.S. hospital in 1939, as she had witnessed it in the South Pacific:

> With all the positive forces at one's disposal—I had enough money, I had knowledge, I had reputation and prestige, I even had a film of a newborn baby in New Guinea to show to the nurses—there are limits to what one can do within a culture. . . . Keeping one's baby in the same hospital room was forbidden by state law. . . . The best that could be done—the closest approximation to rooming-in and self-demand feeding, as these practices later came to be called—was to give me the baby to be fed every three hours.

18. Nestel, "'Other Mothers.'"

19. Goldsmith, *Childbirth Wisdom.*

20. Kitzinger, *Women as Mothers.*

21. Jordan, *Birth in Four Cultures.*

22. Ibid., 1.

23. Natural childbirth proponents protested a variety of childbirth procedures considered routine practice in U.S. hospitals by the 1940s and 1950s. These included shaving the woman's perineum and giving her an enema to "decrease the chance of infection," strapping her arms and legs to the delivery table to avoid "contamination" of the baby (particularly after the use of medications, such as twilight sleep, to which some women reacted violently), performing generous episiotomies to enlarge her vaginal opening, using forceps, and extracting the infant through a vacuum technique. For additional information, see Davis-Floyd, *Birth as an American Rite of Passage,* 83–84, 125–128.

24. Sandelowski, *Pain, Pleasure, and American Childbirth,* 71.

25. Davis-Floyd, *Birth as an American Rite of Passage,* 176–177.

26. Rothman, "Awake and Aware, or False Consciousness"; see also Leavitt, *Brought to Bed,* 214–215.

27. Sullivan and Weitz, *Labor Pains,* 39.

28. Stewart, "Homebirths—A Modern Trend—Is It Progress?"

29. NAPSAC later became the InterNational Association of Parents and Professionals for Safe Alternatives in Childbirth and retained the same acronym.

30. Nelson, "Working-Class Women, Middle-Class Women, and Models of Childbirth," 295.

31. Nestel, "'Other Mothers,'" 8.

32. Leavitt, *Brought to Bed,* 216.

33. De Vries, *Making Midwives Legal,* xiii.

34. For example, Verta Taylor, in "Social Movement Continuity," demonstrates the power of continued feminist organizing between 1945 and 1960. Following the "first-wave" women's movement that some argue culminated in women winning the right to vote in 1920, Taylor suggests that the "second wave" of women's organizing in the 1960s was not an "immaculate conception" of women's activism but an extension of earlier activism (772). See also McCarthy and Zald, "Resource Mobilization and Social Movements," who argue that older movements and organizations also become more effective because of the resources they have both in terms of experience and their constituent base (1233).

35. See Wertz and Wertz, *Lying-In,* 178–190; Klassen, *Blessed Events,* 27–29.

36. Dick-Read, *Childbirth without Fear* and *No Time For Fear.*

37. Klassen, *Blessed Events,* 28. Less charitably, in Richard Wertz and Dorothy Wertz, *Lying-In* (183), they suggest that Grantley Dick-Read "glorified motherhood as a woman's true fulfillment in panegyrics that mixed Victorianism, sentimentality, mysticism, nature philosophy, and religion."

38. Sousa, *Childbirth at Home,* 129; Klassen, *Blessed Events,* 29.

39. Wessel, *Natural Childbirth and the Christian Family*; see also Wertz and Wertz, *Lying-In,* 187.

40. Block, *Pushed!,* 218.

41. Cassidy, *Birth,* 45.

42. Gaskin, *Spiritual Midwifery.*

43. Rooks, *Midwifery and Childbirth in America,* 61.

44. Arms, *Immaculate Deception,* 222; Mehl, "Statistical Outcomes of Homebirth in the U.S.," 77.

45. Reid, "Sisterhood and Professionalization," 226; see also Edwards and Waldorf, *Reclaiming Birth,* 155.

46. Hazell, *Birth Goes Home.*

47. Ibid., 6–8.

48. Ibid., 8.

49. Ruzek, *The Women's Health Movement,* 5.

50. Sandelowski, *Pain, Pleasure, and American Childbirth,* 89.

51. Treichler, "Feminism, Medicine, and the Meaning of Childbirth," 121.

52. Cassidy, *Birth,* 48.

53. National Organization for Women, "1999 NOW Conference Resolutions."

54. Block, *Pushed!,* 270.

55. Nelson, *Women of Color and the Reproductive Rights Movement*; Silliman et al, *Undivided Rights.*

56. Author's field notes, Virginia Birthing Freedom strategy meeting following Joint Commission on Health Care Midwifery Subcommittee hearing, August 6, 1999.

57. Sandelowski, *Pain, Pleasure, and American Childbirth,* 136.

58. De Vries, *Making Midwives Legal,* xi.

59. Edwards and Waldorf, *Reclaiming Birth,* 98.

60. See, for example, Carter, *Come Gently, Sweet Luciana*; Karmel, *Thank You, Dr. Lamaze*; Wessel, *Natural Childbirth and the Christian Family.*

61. Gaskin, *Spiritual Midwifery.*

62. Rich, *Of Woman Born.*

63. Boston Women's Health Collective, *Our Bodies, Ourselves.*

64. Klassen, *Blessed Events*, 59.

65. Nestel, *Obstructed Labour*, 91.

66. Michaelson, *"Childbirth in America,"* 28; see also Rothman, *In Labor* (1991), 94–98.

67. Cosslett, *Women Writing Childbirth*; see, for example, Haire, *The Cultural Warping of Childbirth*; Arms, *Immaculate Deception*; Kitzinger, *Giving Birth*.

68. See, for example, Shaw, *Forced Labor*; Donnison, *Midwives and Medical Men*; Donegan, *Women and Men Midwives*; Ehrenreich and English, *For Her Own Good*; Oakley, *Women Confined*; Scully, *Men Who Control Women's Health*; Rothman, *In Labor* (1982), and *Recreating Motherhood*; Corea, *The Mother Machine*.

69. Boston Women's Health Collective, *Our Bodies, Ourselves*; Gaskin, *Spiritual Midwifery*; Kitzinger, *The Experience of Childbirth*, and *Birth at Home*; Romalis, *Childbirth*.

70. See, for instance, Shanley, *Unassisted Childbirth*; Griesemer, *Unassisted Homebirth*; Halfmoon, *Primal Mothering in a Modern World*.

71. Davis-Floyd, Pigg, and Cosminsky, "Daughters of Time," 106.

72. Debra Susie, *In the Way of Our Grandmothers*, 71–72. Notably, following Susie's study, DEMs also gained licensure in Florida in the early 1990s, a story I revisit later in this chapter.

73. Nelson, "Working-Class Women, Middle-Class Women, and Models of Childbirth"; Lazarus, "What Do Women Want?"

74. Lazarus, "What Do Women Want?" 133.

75. Nelson, "Working-Class Women, Middle-Class Women, and Models of Childbirth," 292.

76. MacDonald, "Tradition as a Political Symbol in the New Midwifery in Canada," 53, emphasis in original.

77. Cosslett, *Women Writing Childbirth*, 9–10; see also Nestel's insightful critique of the presentation of race in depictions of "primitive," "traditional," and "tribal" births in "'Other Mothers.'"

78. Arms, *Immaculate Deception*, 2.

79. As well as idealizing "primitive" women's childbirth experience, other authors in the natural childbirth movement have relied on the trope of "primitive societies" as savage and violent—a reason Western women should appreciate their more "civilized" forms of childbirth. For instance, Sheila Kitzinger, a social anthropologist well known for her advocacy of midwives and homebirth, explained in *The Experience of Childbirth*: "In primitive societies a woman with . . . difficulty [in labor] might find a fire lit on her abdomen to smoke the baby out, or be beaten with sticks to force the child to emerge, or have to confess adultery, which is considered a barrier to spontaneous delivery. We have a good deal to be grateful for in modern Western obstetrics!" (163). Ultimately, she makes no mention—here or elsewhere in the book—of *which* "primitive societies" held such views or engaged in such practices, nor does she offer any additional cultural context for these practices. See also Nestel's critique in "'Other Mothers,'" 10–11.

80. Goldsmith, *Childbirth Wisdom*, 21.

81. Macari, *She Births*, 4, emphasis and spacing in original.

82. Ibid., 136–148. Compare, for instance, Lazarus, "What Do Women Want?" and Davis-Floyd, *Birth as an American Rite of Passage*. Scholars have continued to docu-

ment uncritical connections to a romantic, idealized past within contemporary efforts to support midwives. For instance, Nestel opens her recent book *Obstructed Labour* on Canada's midwifery movement with an anecdote about a nonaboriginal Canadian midwife's attempt to "reclaim" connections with First Nations' "culture and spirit." At a conference to support aboriginal health programs, the midwife advocated that aboriginal women should reject "the white man's institutions" and return "to the way *our* ancestors did it" (emphasis in original speech). Nestel argues that claiming a unified, collective history ultimately ignores "the ways in which white women both benefit from race privilege and have participated in racial dominance" (ibid., 1).

83. Biggs, "Rethinking the History," 32; see also Nestel, "'Other Mothers.'"

84. Romalis, *Childbirth*, 9.

85. Nelson, "Working-Class Women, Middle-Class Women, and Models of Childbirth," 285.

86. Bobel, *The Paradox of Natural Mothering*.

87. Michie and Cahn, "Unnatural Births," 55.

88. See Davis-Floyd, *Birth as an American Rite of Passage*, for a groundbreaking discussion of this process.

89. Sawicki, *Disciplining Foucault*, 82; Foucault, *The History of Sexuality*, 135ff.

90. Rothman, *In Labor* (1982), 79. As Richard Wertz and Dorothy Wertz explain in *Lying-In* (181), in the 1940s, many doctors considered epidural anesthesia, which numbs the lower half of the body, "the answer for women who desired a 'natural childbirth,'" since it allowed them to remain conscious for labor and birth.

91. See also Cassidy, *Birth*, 2.

92. Halfmoon, *Primal Mothering*, 2–3.

93. Block, *Pushed!*, xvii.

94. Pasveer and Akrich, "Obstetrical Trajectories," 236.

95. MacDonald, *At Work in the Field of Birth*, 125.

96. Miller, "Public Argument and Legislative Debate in the Rhetorical Construction of Public Policy"; the Big Push for Midwives, "The Push States." For more detailed information regarding the recent history and the specifics of licensure and regulations for DEMs in the United States, see Rooks, *Midwifery and Childbirth in America*, especially chap. 9; and Davis-Floyd and Johnson, *Mainstreaming Midwifery.* Thank you also to Katie Prown, the campaign manager for the Big Push for Midwives, for helping me clarify this section on the legal status and regulations for DEMs.

97. Sullivan and Weitz, *Labor Pains*, 107; De Vries, *Making Midwives Legal*, xiii; Baer, *Biomedicine and Alternative Healing Systems in America*, 116.

98. De Vries, *Making Midwives Legal*, 175.

99. Rooks, *Midwifery and Childbirth in America*, 241.

100. Citizens for Midwifery, "What Is CfM?"

101. Klassen, *Blessed Events*, 31–32.

102. Klaus, Kennell, and Klaus, *The Doula Book*, 4.

103. Block, *Pushed!*, 156.

104. Cassidy, *Birth*, 196.

105. Block, *Pushed!*, 154.

106. MotherBirth, "Frequently Asked Questions about Doulas."

107. Weisman, *Women's Health Care*, 116; see also Brown, *Prenatal Care*; Horton, *The Women's Health Data Book.*

108. Miller, "Public Argument and Legislative Debate," 367; citing Trunzo, "Children"; Warshaw, "The American Way of Birth"; McNurlin, "Giving Birth"; Heiligman, "The Birthing Center Experience."

109. Davis-Floyd, Pigg, and Cosminsky, "Daughters of Time," 106.

110. Berino, "The History of Direct-Entry Midwifery in Florida," speech (cited in ibid., 106).

111. Mathews, "Killing the Medical Self-Help Tradition among African Americans," 74–75.

112. Fraser, "Afro-American Midwives, Biomedicine and the State," 447.

113. Declerq, Paine, and Winter, "Home Birth in the United States, 1989–1992," 480; see also Schlenzka, "Safety of Alternative Approaches to Childbirth." It is important to note, however, that contemporary demographic data regarding homebirthers are unavoidably fragmentary, primarily because of the unwillingness of many homebirth parents to disclose their attendant for fear of legal action against their midwives in many areas and fear of exposing their own childbirth practices to government surveillance; see Rooks, *Midwifery and Childbirth in America*, 147; Klassen, *Blessed Events*, 19. Acknowledging those limitations, the study by Declerq, Paine, and Winter also suggests that homebirthers are more likely to be older, to start their prenatal care later, to receive fewer prenatal tests (such as ultrasound and amniocentesis), to have a second or subsequent child, to be married, and are less likely to smoke and drink during pregnancy than women birthing in hospitals.

114. Declerq, Paine, and Winter, "Home Birth in the United States," 480.

115. Parker, "Ethnic Differences in Midwife-Attended US Births," 1139.

116. Ibid., 1140.

117. Ibid.

118. De Vries, *Making Midwives Legal*; Baer, *Biomedicine.*

119. Klassen, *Blessed Events*, 20; see also Nelson, "Working-Class Women, Middle-Class Women, and Models of Childbirth"; Lazarus, "What Do Women Want?"; Ruzek, Olesen, and Clarke, *Women's Health*; Whiteford, "Political Economy, Gender, and the Social Production of Health and Illness"; Williams, "Babies and Banks."

120. Fraser, *African American Midwifery in the South* (103); see also Holmes, "African American Midwives in the South," 287. Even to the present, Dennis Brown and Pamela Toussaint's childbirth education book *Mama's Little Baby* notes that African American women who have homebirths swear by them, but that many African American women, "influenced by parents and grandparents who worked hard to give us a better life, still consider giving birth at home 'going backward'" (94).

121. Borst, *Catching Babies*, 44.

122. Indeed, state and medical officials reserved some of their harshest critiques for African American and immigrant midwives during the early twentieth century. In 1916, prominent physician Joseph B. DeLee referred to midwives as "relics of barbarism [practicing in] crowded communities of foreigners." In 1926, Mississippi's director of the Board of Health, Felix Underwood, wrote that African American midwives were "filthy and ignorant and not far removed from the jungles of Africa"; see DeLee, "Progress toward Ideal Obstetrics," 412; Underwood, "Development of Midwifery in Mississippi," 683.

CHAPTER 3: MIDWIVES IN VIRGINIA

1. For a more detailed history of midwives and homebirth mothers in Virginia, see the cultural history I wrote for Virginia midwifery supporters in 2003, now available at www.vabirthpac.org/historyofmidwifery.pdf.

2. Fraser, *African American Midwifery in the South,* 11.

3. Fraser, *African American Midwifery in the South,* 59–60.

4. Plecker, "Virginia Makes Efforts to Solve Midwife Problem," 809.

5. E. R. Hardin, "The Midwife Problem," 347.

6. Plecker, "Virginia Makes Efforts."

7. Echoing national trends, women of color and poor women fared especially poorly during the forced eugenic sterilization campaign in Virginia, when over 8,000 women whom the state deemed defective were sterilized between 1924 and 1979; see Lombardo, "Eugenic Sterilization in Virginia"; P. Hardin, "Eugenics Affected Va. Law," A13.

8. Fraser, *African American Midwifery in the South,* 75.

9. P. Hardin, "'Documentary Genocide.'" In his 1943 letter to local registrars, physicians, health officers, nurses, school superintendents, and clerks of the courts entitled "Surnames by Counties and Cities, Virginia Families Striving to Pass as 'Indian' and/or White," Walter Plecker argued:

> Now that these people are playing up the advantages gained by being permitted to give "Indian" as the race of the child's parents on birth certificates, we see the great mistake made in not stopping earlier the organized propagation of this racial falsehood. They have been using the advantage thus gained as an aid to intermarriage into the white race and to attend white schools, and now for some time they have been refusing to register with war draft boards as negroes. . . . Some of these mongrels, finding that they have been able to sneak in their birth certificates unchallenged as Indians are now making a rush to register as white. . . . One hundred and fifty thousand other mulattoes in Virginia are watching eagerly the attempt of their pseudo-Indian brethren, ready to follow in a rush when the first have made a break in the dike.

Plecker's mandate to reclassify "Indians" as "Negroes" remained in effect until the racial integrity laws were repealed in 1975. Thus, as "Negroes," American Indian women were also at higher risk of eugenic sterilization in Virginia, as indicated in the Virginia Sterilization Act of 1924, which was passed in connection with the Racial Integrity Act; see P. Hardin, "Eugenics Affected Va. Law." The Virginia Sterilization Act was not repealed until 1979; see Baskervill, "House Panel Approves Apology for Eugenics."

10. P. Hardin, "'Documentary Genocide,'" A10.

11. Fraser, *African American Midwifery in the South,* 72.

12. Ibid., 63.

13. "Midwifery Manual," 6–7, reproduced in Smith and Roberson, *My Bag Was Always Packed,* 155.

14. Virginia State Board of Health, "Midwife Instruction."

15. Bennett, "Midwife Work in Virginia," 526.

16. Fraser, *African American Midwifery in the South*, 209–210; Gwynne Jenkins has noted a similar phenomenon in Costa Rica, where midwives' feelings of alienation from both legislative efforts to curtail their practice and the rejection of the homebirth model by women in their communities—and thus midwives' expertise—led to their retirement. See Jenkins, "Burning Bridges."

17. Fraser, *African American Midwifery in the South*, 86, 131.

18. Ibid., 132.

19. Lombardo, "Eugenic Sterilization in Virginia"; P. Hardin, "Eugenics Affected Va. Law."

20. Baughman, "A Preliminary Report upon the Midwife Situation in Virginia," 749.

21. Commonwealth of Virginia, Department of Health, Center for Health Statistics, as cited in Commonwealth of Virginia, Joint Commission on Health Care (hereafter cited as JCHC), "Summary of Public Comments," 4.

22. Fraser, *African American Midwifery in the South*, 95.

23. Even as African Americans were admitted to Virginia hospitals in larger numbers during the mid-1900s, they still faced segregation in childbirth clinics until the passage of the Civil Rights Act in 1964. For example, the largest public hospital, the Medical College of Virginia Hospital in Richmond (MCV), had a separate building for African Americans, the St. Phillips Hospital, until 1965. Even after the official end of segregated hospital care, in her memoir with Roberson, *Memories of a Black Lay Midwife from Northern Neck Virginia,* Smith recalls one African American woman's reaction to the persistence of "separate" waiting rooms: "Doctors then had two waiting rooms. . . . I knew one woman in her twenties who said it made her so mad that she intentionally sat on the side where everybody else was waiting. She said that people stared at her like she was in the wrong place and she shouldn't be there, that was in 1980" (24).

24. Fraser, *African American Midwifery in the South*, 88.

25. Smith and Roberson, *Memories of a Black Lay Midwife*, 23.

26. Fraser, *African American Midwifery in the South*, 157; Smith and Roberson, *My Bag Was Always Packed*, 26.

27. Jones, "Will There Be a Place for Nurse Midwives?" 173.

28. Smith and Roberson, *My Bag Was Always Packed*, 120–121.

29. Stern, "A Public Health Perspective on Midwifery by the Director of the Office of Family Health Services," 4.

30. JCHC, "Midwifery Study," 2.

31. Stevens, *In Sickness and in Wealth,* 175, 254; Smith and Roberson, *My Bag Was Always Packed*, 46.

32. Susie, *In the Way of Our Grandmothers,* viii, cited in Smith and Roberson, *My Bag Was Always Packed*, 115.

33. JCHC, "Midwifery Study," 3. The American College of Nurse-Midwifery was incorporated in 1955. In 1969, the American Association of Nurse-Midwives merged with the American College of Nurse-Midwifery to form the American College of Nurse-Midwives (ACNM), as it is currently called; see the ACNM website, www.midwife.org/about/history.cfm.

34. Commonwealth of Virginia, *The Code of Virginia*, §32.1–145.

35. My interviews with women utilizing and/or offering midwifery services during the 1970s indicate that most were unaware of the passage of this legislation. In fact,

some midwives, both in rural and urban areas, continued to provide homebirth services well into the 1990s before becoming aware that their practice was a criminal offense when midwives began to be investigated by the state.

36. Ibid., §32.1–145.

37. JCHC, "Midwifery Study," 4.

38. Ibid.

39. The last legally permitted lay midwife in Virginia was Adella Scott Wilson, who assisted in approximately 2,000 births in the Virginia Beach area during her thirty-four years of practice; see Forster, "Welcome Home," A4.

40. American College of Nurse-Midwives, "State by State Chart of Laws and Regulations That Need to Be Changed."

41. Commonwealth of Virginia, *The Code of Virginia*, §54.1–2901.

42. Commonwealth of Virginia, Department of Health Professions and Virginia Health Planning Board, Task Force on the Study of Obstetric Access and Certified Nurse-Midwives (hereafter cited as Task Force), "The Potential for Expansion of the Practice of Nurse Midwives," 20.

43. Heneghan, "They've Come a Long Way, Baby, Midwives," 34.

44. Ibid., 33; Task Force, "The Potential for Expansion of the Practice of Nurse Midwives," iv; American College of Nurse-Midwives (2000), "Certified Nurse-Midwives in Virginia."

45. Heneghan, "They've Come a Long Way," 33.

46. American College of Nurse-Midwives (2000), "Certified Nurse-Midwives in Virginia."

47. American College of Nurse-Midwives (2008), "Certified Nurse-Midwives in Virginia."

48. Forster, "Welcome Home," A4.

49. Author's transcription, Presentation to the Board of Medicine, August 3, 2001. Due to the tenuous legal situation for midwives in Virginia during much of my fieldwork, I identify speakers by real names only when quoting public discourse, such as comments credited in newspaper articles and from public presentations (such as those made during legislative or judicial hearings). Some of these speakers also participated in my research through interviews, though many did not.

50. Task Force, "The Potential for Expansion of the Practice of Nurse Midwives," 10.

51. JCHC, "Midwifery Study," 5.

52. Ibid.

53. Heneghan, "They've Come a Long Way," 33.

54. BirthCare and Women's Health's, "BirthCare's History." Prior to my fieldwork, I worked briefly as an administrative assistant at BirthCare in 1998.

55. Ibid.

56. van Olphen-Fehr, *Diary of a Midwife*, 103.

57. Strobel, "Going Back to the Roots, Midwives," 27–28.

58. Ibid.

59. Pegram, "Unlicensed Midwives Can't Practice Legally under Virginia Statute," B5.

60. Newby, as cited in Norris, "Birthrites," 74.

61. Pegram, "Unlicensed Midwives Can't Practice," B5.

62. Glod and White, "Midwives Charged in Death of Va. Woman," B1; Neuberger, "Traditional Midwife Extols Value, Rewards She Discovered," A1.

63. Ibid.

64. Ibid. To the excitement of many midwifery supporters, Hughes received her license and began to practice again in Virginia following the 2005 legislation to license CPMs.

65. Author's field notes, plea bargain hearing, May 5, 2000.

66. Voices for Healthcare Rights Fund, "Stafford Case against Midwives Unravels amidst New Questions," press release, May 2, 2000.

67. Neuberger, "Officials Explain Charges against Two Midwives," B1. As Kiran Krishnamurthy explains in "Midwife Expected to Enter Guilty Plea," B4, critics of the prosecution also questioned the impartiality of Chief State Medical Examiner Marcella Fierro, who was married to a Richmond obstetrician and vocally opposed the licensure of DEMs. I first encountered Fierro when she reported to lawmakers at a Health, Welfare, and Institutions Subcommittee meeting regarding the licensure of DEMs in 2001, "We do see, each year, a few deaths where there was no physician involved, where the woman, generally it is due to postpartum hemorrhage, where this has not been recognized and the woman has been allowed to bleed for hours and hours and hours and then dies of shock" (author's transcription, January 30, 2001). Following a legislator's request for specific statistics regarding maternal deaths as a result of homebirths with midwives, Fierro was unable to substantiate her claims, repeating several times, "We don't have figures for that" (author's transcription, January 30, 2001).

68. Greenspun became well known a few years later as the lead lawyer for John Allen Mohammed, the sniper who killed ten people in the Washington, D.C., area in 2002.

69. Krishnamurthy, "Unlicensed Midwives Get Jail Sentences," A1.

70. Hall, "Death and Its Consequences"; Glod and White, "Midwives Charged in Death of Va. Woman," B1.

71. According to Gertrude Fraser, in *African American Midwifery in the South*, during the early 1900s, midwives in Virginia could have their permits revoked for "entering the birth canal" (153). A "Midwife Manual" from the Virginia State Department of Health in the mid-1900s, which reviewed safety rules for midwives, read: "Rule Three: She must not pass her fingers or any instrument into the birth canal of the woman, for the purpose of making an examination or for any other purpose," as reproduced in Smith and Roberson, *My Bag Was Always Packed*, 155. This set up a historical precedent for internal examinations to constitute the "practice of medicine" in Virginia, which is a crime often prosecuted as a felony.

72. Claire Peters, an intensive-care nurse, was present at Julia Peters's birth and assisted EMTs in their attempts to resuscitate her daughter-in-law. She was charged with perjury in connection to her testimony before a Secret Grand Jury, though her case was dropped following Cynthia Caillagh's guilty plea.

73. Callaigh, press release, May 5, 2000.

74. Block, *Pushed!*, 218–248.

75. Voices for Healthcare Rights Fund, "Stafford Case against Midwives Unravels," press release, May 2, 2000. Commonwealth of Virginia, *The Code of Virginia*, §18.2–369.

76. In particular, Rachel Roth highlights how "fetal rights" arguments, stemming from anti-abortion efforts, have ultimately—if largely unintentionally—made pregnant women more vulnerable to state and medical intervention during pregnancy because what the state deems the safety of the fetus can legally trump a woman's right to make decisions about her health and healthcare during her pregnancy; see Roth, *Making Women Pay*, 97.

77. Hall, "The Decision, Cradle and Grave," "Labor and Delivery," "The Descent," "The Midwife," "Death and Its Consequences."

78. Voices for Healthcare Rights Fund, "Alternative Healthcare Practitioners," press release, 1999. Krishnamurthy, "Midwife Expected to Enter Guilty Plea," B4. Contributing to Caillagh and Elizabeth Haw supporters' discontent, prosecuting attorney Eric Olson later thanked reporter Jim Hall in court for his investigative contributions to the prosecution's case (author's field notes, plea bargain hearing, May 5, 2000).

79. Author's field notes, plea bargain hearing, May 5, 2000.

80. Krishnamurthy, "Unlicensed Midwives Get Jail Sentences," A1.

81. Neuberger, "Traditional Midwife Extols Value," A1.

82. Wagner, "A Modern-Day Witch Hunt in Virginia," A13.

83. Goodman, "Trial Outcome."

84. The increasing urbanization of all CNM practices in Virginia—particularly those CNMs who offered homebirth services—ran counter to the initial state and medical support of midwives to serve rural and medically underserved areas; see, for example, Task Force, "The Potential for the Expansion of the Practice of Nurse Midwives." However, the migration of obstetricians from "rural areas [in Virginia] because of heavy workloads and little financial gain" left a dearth of prenatal care and delivery services by both physicians and CNMs; see Davis-Floyd, *Birth as an American Right of Passage*, 300; see also Governor's Work Group on Rural Obstetrical Care, "Executive Directive 2: Report of the Governor's Work Group on Rural Obstetrical Care."

85. JCHC, "Midwifery Study," 5.

86. Greene, "Information Sheet," 1.

87. Commonwealth of Virginia, "Study; direct-entry midwifery."

88. In 1999, midwifery proponents also worked to introduce identical bills to the House of Delegates and Senate Rules Committee, which would have registered and permitted lay midwives under the regulations set forth prior to 1977. These bills were briefly reviewed, but no action was taken in the House, and the Senate struck the bill from the docket.

89. For a discussion of the complicated politics surrounding such decisions, see De Vries, *Making Midwives Legal*.

90. Virginia Midwifery Coalition Listserv message, Brynne Potter, 2000. Potter is a homebirth mother and was a seasoned organizer around a variety of progressive causes when she organized the VMC. She ultimately became a CPM and served as the primary representative of the Commonwealth Midwives Alliance during efforts to legalize CPMs between 2003 and 2005.

91. Hughes and Wood, "Information Sheet for Commonwealth Midwives Alliance."

92. As reported in JCHC, "Midwifery Study," 8–9. In 1998, ACNM began to certify midwives as certified midwives (CMs); these practitioners do not have a nursing

degree, but other aspects and standards of their education and examinations remain commensurate with CNMs.

CHAPTER 4: MOTHERS IN THE LEGISLATURE

1. Baer, *Biomedicine and Alternative Healing Systems in America*; Morgen, *Into Our Own Hands*, 130.

2. See, for example, Litoff, *American Midwives* and *The American Midwifery Debate*; Lay, *The Rhetoric of Midwifery*; Miller, "Public Argument and Legislative Debate in the Rhetorical Construction of Public Policy."

3. Nestel, *Obstructed Labour*, 83.

4. Solinger, *Pregnancy and Power*.

5. Foucault, *Discipline and Punish*, 184.

6. Davis-Floyd, *Birth as an American Rite of Passage*, 152.

7. This strategy was heavily debated on Listservs prior to legislative hearings. As noted, proponents felt that the presence of children would portray these mothers as "respectable." Opponents, however, argued that bringing children took away from the "professional" image that homebirth mothers aimed to portray. See also Nestel's discussion of "visible respectability" among midwives in *Obstructed Labour*, 100, 106–108.

8. Abraham Lincoln, "Gettysburg Address," November 19, 1863.

9. Commonwealth of Virginia, Joint Commission on Health Care (hereafter cited as JCHC), "Midwifery Study," 8.

10. Gerheart, "Joint Commission on Health Care to Study Lay Midwives and Obstetrical Education in Med Schools," 2.

11. Murray, "Direct Entry Midwifery Study by Senior Health Policy Analyst for the Joint Commission on Health Care," 10, and "Staff Follow-up from Last Meeting by Senior Health Policy Analyst for the Joint Commission on Health Care," 5.

12. JCHC, "Summary of Public Comments," 1–2.

13. Ibid., 3. The subcommittee also received twenty-three written public comments from individuals and organizations, twenty-two of which supported the legalization of midwifery.

14. The Joint Commission on Health Care's final report to the governor and General Assembly of Virginia, the "Midwifery Study," 21, read:

> A more subjective observation is that the current state law provides a disincentive for persons receiving direct entry midwifery services to seek medical attention when such attention is warranted. It should be noted that the practice of direct entry midwifery is currently illegal, but the receipt of such services is not. Nevertheless, the current illegal status of direct entry midwifery could delay persons from seeking medical attention for a mother and her baby when necessary, when the desirable public policy goal would be to have such services sought as quickly as possible. A further subjective observation is that parents who chose direct entry midwifery services appear to be highly motivated to do so, and it is unclear that the desire to seek such services is influenced significantly, if at all, by the legal status of direct entry midwifery.
>
> It should be further noted that the public policy decision against the practice of direct entry midwifery during the 1976 session of the General Assem-

bly was clouded by the General Assembly's decision to grandfather existing practitioners. There is one direct entry midwife still legally and actively practicing today, as she has been since 1972, with the full impirateur [sic] of the state. Therefore it is difficult to cogently argue that the public policy position of the state is that direct entry midwifery is patently unsafe. If this were the case, then there would have been no justification for the grandfathering provisions included in 1976.

15. The American College of Nurse-Midwives, as discussed in Chapters 2 and 3, also certifies certified midwives (CMs), who take the same certification exam as students of nurse-midwifery programs but do not have a nursing degree. The CM certification was not seriously considered in Virginia after initial mention by CNMs in 1998 and 1999 in part because CMs were legally recognized only in New York at that time (New York began licensing CMs in 1992). Rhode Island revised its CNM rules and regulations to include the CM in 2000 (the first CM was licensed in 2004 and, at the time of publication, she was the only person to have requested licensure in Rhode Island). New Jersey adopted CM certification in 2003. Thank you to Ronnie Lichtman, Linda Nanni, and Michelle Palmer for their assistance with these dates.

16. North American Registry of Midwives, "North American Registry of Midwives Mission Statement."

17. Davis-Floyd, "The Ups, Downs, and Interlinkages of Nurse- and Direct-Entry Midwifery."

18. North American Registry of Midwives, "CPM Brochure Text."

19. During the JCHC hearings in 1999 and 2000 to study DEMs, representatives of VA-ACOG reiterated the American College of Obstetricians and Gynecologist's statement of policy on homebirth, which was initially drafted in 1979:

> Labor and delivery, while a physiologic process, clearly presents potential hazards to mother and fetus before and after birth. These hazards require standards of safety which are provided in the hospital setting and cannot be matched in the home situation.
>
> We support those actions that improve the experience of the family while continuing to provide the mother and her infant with accepted standards of safety available only in hospitals which conform to the standards as outlined by the American Academy of Pediatricians and the American College of Obstetricians and Gynecologists. (Cited in JCHC, "Midwifery Study," 9).

20. Heyser, "Midwifery Expansion Fails as Proposal from Health Panel," B2.

21. See, for example, Cruikshank, *The Will to Empower*; Edwards, "The Social Control of Illegitimacy through Adoption"; Hyatt, "Poverty and the Medicalisation of Motherhood"; Lopez, "Agency and Constraint"; Morgen, "'It's the Whole Power of the City against Us!'"; Whiteford, "Political Economy, Gender, and the Social Production of Health and Illness"; Williams, "Babies and Banks."

22. Michel Foucault has called the discourses and practices that surveil and control individual bodies—and thus entire populations—"bio-power," which he argues is "an indispensable element in the development of capitalism." See *The History of Sexuality,* 140–141; see also Sawicki, *Disciplining Foucault,* 67–68. Although Foucault never

addressed the disciplining of women's bodies through medical and state surveillance of pregnancy, birth, and mothering, he explained the collusion of medicine and politics under capitalism more broadly in his lecture "The Birth of Social Medicine," 137:

> Capitalism, which developed from the end of the eighteenth century to the beginning of the nineteenth century, started by socializing a first object, the body, as a factor of productive [and, I would add, reproductive] force, of labor power. Society's control over individuals was accomplished not only through consciousness or ideology but also in the body and with the body. For capitalist society, it was biopolitics, the biological, the somatic, the corporeal, that mattered more than anything else. The body is a biopolitical reality; medicine is a biopolitical strategy.

23. Ward, *La Leche League*, 37.

24. The medical lobby is powerful in a variety of ways in Virginia (similar to its national prominence). Many physicians are socially involved with lawmakers, and the healthcare industry is one of the most substantial financial contributors to lawmakers' campaigns. According to the Virginia Public Access Project (VPAP), the "Health Care Industry" was the largest candidate donor industry in Virginia in 2000, the second largest in 2001, and the third largest in 2002 (personal communication, David M. Poole, executive director of VPAP, September 4, 2003). There was no record of campaign contributions by midwifery advocacy groups during this time.

25. Author's transcription of John Partridge, Health, Welfare, and Institutions (HWI) Committee meeting, February 8, 2000. Unless otherwise noted, the transcriptions of meetings are my own, with assistance from Asan Askin, Janet Gallay, Anna Inazu, Robbie Kaplan, and Emily Tumpson. I use the following transcription conventions throughout the rest of this chapter:

> [brackets] indicate text inserted for clarity
> /backslashes/ indicate unclear portions of recording; transcription
>   is based on field notes
> (text) within parentheses indicates the actions of the speaker, such as
>   (laughing)
> . . . indicates a pause by the speaker
> . . . . indicates the omission of text by the author
> text- indicates a word that was abruptly cut off by the speaker
> *italics* in the body of the text indicate excerpts from transcribed
>   testimony or interviews

26. Martin, *The Woman in the Body*, 56; Rothman, *Recreating Motherhood*, 55–57, 171.

27. Jordan, "Authoritative Knowledge and Its Construction," 57.

28. Ironically, in a later Senate Education and Health Subcommittee meeting in the Virginia General Assembly in 2000, a delegate asked another representative of VA-ACOG, "Do you have any evidence showing that homebirth is unsafe or that midwives aren't practicing safely in other states?" The physician looked flustered and replied, "No, no evidence"; see Hamblet, "Views of a Homebirth Advocate," 12.

29. Sawicki, *Disciplining Foucault*, 67–68.

30. Jordan, "Authoritative Knowledge," 56.

31. Roth, *Making Women Pay*.

32. Simonds, Rothman, and Norman, *Laboring On*, 199.

33. Klassen, *Blessed Events*, 61.

34. Two of the three female physicians who spoke in opposition to bills in 2000, 2001, and 2002 mentioned their status as mothers, while none of the six male speakers acknowledged any connections to fatherhood.

35. Author's transcription, Anne Peterson, HWI Committee meeting, January 30, 2001.

36. The presentation of homebirth as a challenge to American values has historical precedence in the United States. For example, Stanley Lemons notes in *The Woman Citizen*, 159–166, that physicians arguing against the training of midwives under the Sheppard-Towner Maternal and Infancy Protection Act in the 1920s also suggested that the "socialization" of American medicine was indeed un-American. See, for example Mabbott's 1907 invective against midwives in "The Regulation of Midwives in New York." As Neal Devitt has suggested in "The Statistical Case for Elimination of the Midwife," "Obstetricians were engaged in something more than a public-spirited campaign to lower infant and maternal mortality" (89). Later, in 1962, Waldo Fielding and Lois Benjamin, in *The Childbirth Challenge*, denounced the un-American origins of natural childbirth techniques in Europe and the Soviet Union as threats to democracy and womanhood in America. In contrast, in 1957 National Childbirth Trust directors Prunella Briance and Grantley Dick Read, in Briance, *Natural Childbirth*, made appeals to Britain as "the mother country" to adopt a more enlightened approach to birth: "Babies born this way [without anesthesia, in the home, and/or by midwives] are better babies . . . and we urgently need in Britain a race of good quality men and women" (quoted in Kitzinger, "Strategy of the Early Childbirth Movement," 99). Clearly, nationalistic values around childbirth can, and have, functioned as flexible political tools.

37. Fraser, *African American Midwifery in the South*, 132.

38. Ibid., 86.

39. Declerq, Paine, and Winter, "Home Birth in the United States, 1989–1992," 480.

40. As cited in Forster, "Welcome Home," A1.

41. In 2002, midwifery supporters strategized with supportive delegates and lobbyists to introduce three bills to regulate DEMs: for license as CPMs, for Virginia to support its own certification and licensure of midwives, and for Virginia to merely require midwives to obtain permits from the state to practice. Their strategy was to be flexible regarding requirements, allowing legislators to choose which option was most viable within the existing healthcare system and ultimately to pass only one.

42. Author's transcription, Steven Bentheim, HWI Committee meeting, January 24, 2002.

43. Hyatt, "Poverty and the Medicalisation of Motherhood," 103.

44. Author's field notes, Joint Commission on Health Care Midwifery Subcommittee hearing, August 6, 1999.

45. Fraser, *African American Midwifery in the South*; Gordon, *Pitied but Not Entitled*; Whiteford, "Political Economy;" Hyatt, "Poverty."

46. Whiteford, "Political Economy," 249; see also Nelson, *Women of Color and the Reproductive Rights Movement*, 183.

47. Foucault, *The History of Sexuality*; Sawicki, *Disciplining Foucault*.

48. Author's transcription, Ellen Hamblet, HWI Committee meeting, January 30, 2001.

49. Author's transcription, Ellen Hamblet, HWI Committee meeting, February 8, 2000.

50. Author's transcription, Ellen Hamblet, HWI Committee Meeting, January 24, 2002.

51. Virginia Birthing Freedom Listserv message, Ellen Hamblet, 2000

52. Author's transcription, Robert McBride, Senate Committee on Education and Health hearing, February 24, 2004.

53. Author's transcription, Janet Howell, Senate Committee on Education and Health hearing, February 24, 2004.

54. A handful of obstetricians attended homebirths in Virginia into the late 1900s. In this case, the senator described the pro-homebirth obstetrician as "very avant-garde."

55. CNMs also lobbied successfully for legislation to change supervision requirements in 2006, which has loosened restrictions on physician supervision in some rural areas. Many hope that future legislation will expand CNMs' ability to practice autonomously throughout the state.

CHAPTER 5: "I'M NOT REALLY POLITICALLY ACTIVE, BUT . . ."

1. See, for example, Bookman and Morgen, *Women and the Politics of Empowerment*; Lamphere, Zavella, and Gonzales, with Evans, *Sunbelt Working Mothers*; Naples, *Grassroots Warriors*; Goode, "Let's Get Our Act Together"; Hyatt, "From Citizen to Volunteer."

2. Morgen, "'It's the Whole Power of the City against Us!'" 111, emphases in original.

3. Naples, *Grassroots Warriors*, 12.

4. See especially Bookman and Morgen, *Women and the Politics of Empowerment*; Naples, *Grassroots Warriors*.

5. Naples, *Grassroots Warriors*, 111.

6. Bookman and Morgen, *Women and the Politics of Empowerment*, 13.

7. Ibid., 11.

8. Naples, *Grassroots Warriors*, 125.

9. Personal interview, Evie Diaz, 2001. Unless otherwise noted, the transcriptions of interviews are my own, with assistance from Asan Askin, Janet Gallay, Anna Inazu, Robbie Kaplan, and Emily Tumpson. Pseudonyms are used to protect the identity of all participants. I use first rather than last names after participants' initial introduction because this was how both midwives and midwifery supporters preferred to be known in their communities. I use the following transcription conventions throughout the rest of this chapter:

> [brackets] indicate text inserted for clarity
>
> /backslashes/ indicate unclear portions of recording; transcription
> is based on field notes
>
> (text) within parentheses indicates the actions of the speaker,
> such as (laughing)

... indicates a pause by the speaker

.... indicates the omission of text by the author

text- indicates a word that was abruptly cut off by the speaker

italics in the body of the text indicate excerpts from transcribed
       testimony or interviews

10. Personal interview, Uzella Kendall, 2002.

11. Personal interview, Anna Turner, 2002.

12. Personal interview, Fern Jackson, 2002.

13. Personal interview, Greta Davis, 2001.

14. Personal interview, Theresa Neal, 2001.

15. See also Martin, *The Woman in the Body*; Davis-Floyd, *Birth as an American Rite of Passage*; Kahn, *Bearing Meaning*; Hyatt, "From Citizen to Volunteer."

16. Personal interview, Cindy Newton, 2002.

17. Personal interview, Paula Queen, 2002.

18. Lopez, "Agency and Constraint," 160.

19. Personal interview, Evie Diaz, 2001.

20. See also Hyatt, "From Citizen to Volunteer," for a broader discussion of women as volunteers under neoliberalism.

21. Brown, *Replacing Citizenship*, 85.

22. Personal interview, Nancy Davis, 2001.

23. Personal interview, Cindy Newton, 2002.

24. Ibid.

25. Krauss, "Women of Color on the Front Line," 263–264.

26. Personal interview, Zora White, 2002.

27. Ibid.

28. Although women throughout the country elect to have "unattended" homebirths (also called "unassisted" or DIY [do-it-yourself] homebirths), without trained practitioners in attendance (see www.unassistedhomebirth.com), this trend grew dramatically in Virginia in the 1990s, when midwives were forced to stop practicing in many areas.

29. Personal interview, unnamed participant, 2002.

30. Personal interview, Jackie Grayson, 2002.

31. Personal interview, Dera Haviland, 2002.

32. Personal interview, Elsa Harden, 2002.

33. Shanley and Breen-Rothman, "Freebirth Movement"; Block, *Pushed!*, 101.

34. Hatch, as quoted in an online book review of Griesemer, *Unassisted Homebirth*; see also, Halfmoon, *Primal Mothering in a Modern World*, 7.

35. See also Katz, "Childbirth and the Law."

36. See Lapp, "The Home-Birth Controversy."

37. Schor, *The Overspent American*, 136.

38. Bobel, *The Paradox of Natural Mothering*, 119.

39. Ibid., 152, emphasis in original.

40. Personal interview, Val Coleman, 2001.

41. Personal interview, Gaia Riverton, 2002.

42. Bobel, *The Paradox of Natural Mothering*, 144.

43. Personal interview, Dera Haviland, 2002.

44. Virginia Birthing Freedom Listserv message, Terri Jacobs, 2000.

45. Personal interview, Evie Diaz, 2001.

46. Personal interview, Crystal Roberts, 2002.

47. For discussion of a similar phenomenon regarding the stark contrast between white midwives' political influence in Canada versus the absence of women of color in political arenas, see Nestel, *Obstructed Labour*, 32.

CHAPTER 6: DIVISIVE STRATEGIES

1. Kingfisher and Maskovsky, "Introduction," 121.

2. The Declaration of Independence of the Thirteen Colonies, July 4, 1776.

3. Evans, *Born for Liberty*, 172.

4. Bambara, *The Black Woman*.

5. See, for example, Taylor, "Social Movement Continuity"; Freedman, "Beyond the Waves."

6. United Nations General Assembly, "Universal Declaration of Human Rights," Article 1.

7. Grewal, *Transnational America*, 121. Although it is beyond the scope of my discussion here, see Inderpal Grewal's chapter in *Transnational America*, "'Women's Rights as Human Rights': The Transnational Production of Global Feminist Subjects," for an incisive critique of how human rights became not only a means of ensuring the rights of individuals but also an "ethical regime," as this terminology assumed primacy in struggles for refugee rights, environmental rights, global citizenship, food security, and healthcare, as well as feminist efforts for women's equality. Grewal argues further that increasingly broad claims to human rights during the second half of the twentieth century ultimately revived colonial relationships and notions of the "white man's burden," particularly as they were deployed to address "international" inequities, but were frequently ignored by activists in countries such as the United States, where "feminists did not resort to claims of human rights violations since it was assumed that they did not lack human rights" (129). As a case in point, reproductive rights first became tied to human rights discourse in the United States not by feminist activists but through the legal case regarding a white man sentenced to sterilization in *Skinner v. Oklahoma*.

8. Morgan and Roberts, "Rights and Reproduction in Latin America," 12.

9. Solinger, *Pregnancy and Power*, 140, emphasis is original.

10. For further discussion of this case, see Solinger, *Pregnancy and Power*, 93–94; Lombardo, "Eugenic Sterilization in Virginia."

11. *Buck v. Bell,* 274 U.S. 200 (1927). Notably, it was not until May 2, 2002, that Virginia Governor Mark Warner publicly apologized for the state's "shameful effort in which state government never should have been involved" on the seventy-fifth anniversary of *Buck v. Bell*; Warner, "Statement of Governor Mark R. Warner on the 75th Anniversary of the *Buck vs. Bell* Decision."

12. Ordover, *American Eugenics*, 135.

13. *Skinner v. Oklahoma*, 316 U.S. 535 (1942).

14. Solinger, *Pregnancy and Power*, 141.

15. Luker, *Abortion and the Politics of Motherhood*, 92–93.

16. Solinger, *Pregnancy and Power*, 180.

17. *Griswold v. Connecticut*, 381 U.S. 479 (1965).

18. *Eisenstadt v. Baird*, 405 U.S. 438 (1972).

19. *Roe v. Wade*, 410 U.S. 113 (1973).

20. Luker, *Abortion and the Politics*, 157.

21. Solinger, *Beggars and Choosers*, 7.

22. Sandel, *Democracy's Discontent*, 222.

23. Cross, *An All-Consuming Century*, 123, 148; Cohen, *A Consumer's Republic*. Writing about the "consumer movement" during the Great Depression of the 1930s, Lizabeth Cohen makes a distinction between what she calls "citizen consumers," those who protected consumer safety and fought for the fair treatment of consumers in the marketplace, and "purchaser consumers," those who contributed "to the larger society more by exercising their purchasing power than through asserting themselves politically" (18–19). I argue that it is this later form of consumer identity that has intensified under neoliberalism, particularly as it has become central to recent activist efforts. As Cohen notes, politicians during the 1980s saw much of the legislation granting consumer protection from monopolies in earlier decades as misguided yet continued to couch their defense of privatization and deregulation "in the old language of serving the consumer interest" (392). Thus activists have increasingly adopted "consumer rights" rhetoric to address their access to various markets, and not protections within them.

24. Nader, "Introduction," x.

25. Cross, *An All-Consuming Century*, 157–158; Solinger, *Beggars and Choosers*, 6.

26. Evans, *Sexual Citizenship*, 5–6.

27. Cruikshank, *The Will to Empower*, 123.

28. Kessler-Harris, *In Pursuit of Equity*, 13.

29. Solinger, *Beggars and Choosers*, 7, emphasis in original.

30. McCarthy and Zald, "Resource Mobilization and Social Movements," 1221–1222.

31. Virginia Birthing Freedom Listserv message, Thomas Danforth, 2000. Pseudonyms are used to protect the identity of all participants. I use first rather than last names after participants' initial introduction because this was how both midwives and midwifery supporters preferred to be known in their communities.

32. Author's transcription, Ellen Hamblet, Health, Welfare, and Institutions Committee meeting, February 8, 2000. Unless otherwise noted, the transcriptions of meetings and interviews are my own, with assistance from Asan Askin, Janet Gallay, Anna Inazu, Robbie Kaplan, and Emily Tumpson. I use the following transcription conventions throughout the rest of this chapter:

> [brackets] indicate text inserted for clarity
>
> /backslashes/ indicate unclear portions of recording; transcription is based on field notes
>
> (text) within parentheses indicates the actions of the speaker, such as (laughing)
>
> . . . indicates a pause by the speaker
>
> . . . . indicates the omission of text by the author
>
> text- indicates a word that was abruptly cut off by the speaker
>
> *italics* in the body of the text indicate excerpts from transcribed testimony or interviews

33. Personal interview, Fern Jackson, 2002.

34. Ibid.

35. Personal interview, unnamed participant, 2002.

36. MacDonald, "Tradition as a Political Symbol in the New Midwifery in Canada," 56.

37. Bourgeault, *Push!*, 67.

38. Personal interview, unnamed participant, 2001.

39. Personal interview, Zora White, 2002.

40. Personal interview, Anna Turner, 2002.

41. Virginia Birthing Freedom Listserv message, Norma Robbins, 2000.

42. Personal interview, Cindy Newton, 2002.

43. Davis-Floyd and Dumit, "Cyborg Babies," 2.

44. Ginsburg and Rapp, *Conceiving the New World Order*.

45. Rapp, *Testing Women, Testing the Fetus*, 168–171.

46. Personal interview, Tara Mason, 2002.

47. Personal interview, Nelly Vicars, 2002.

48. Ruzek, "Rethinking Feminist Ideologies and Actions," 314.

49. Personal interview, Val Coleman, 2001.

50. Personal interview, Nancy Davis, 2001.

51. See also Lazarus, "What Do Women Want?" 133; Nelson, "Working-Class Women, Middle-Class Women, and Models of Childbirth."

52. Personal interview, Kevin Rogers, 2001.

53. Personal interview, Sara Rogers and Kevin Rogers, 2001.

54. Personal interview, Paula Queen, 2002.

55. Personal interview, Jackie Grayson, 2002.

56. Personal interview, Cindy Newton, 2002.

57. Nestel, *Obstructed Labour*, 30.

58. Ibid., 100.

59. Personal interview, Paula Queen, 2002.

60. Personal interview, Sandy Smith, 2002.

61. Personal interview, unnamed participant, 2007. Since I was only able to conduct interviews with six prior participants during my trip to Virginia in 2007 (as well as several new midwives and homebirthers), I have not included names or pseudonyms for follow-up interviews to better maintain the anonymity of these participants.

62. Personal interview, unnamed participant, 2007.

63. Personal interview, unnamed participant, 2007.

64. Solinger, *Beggars and Choosers*, 5.

65. Personal interview, unnamed participant, 2007.

66. Hyatt, "Poverty and the Medicalisation of Motherhood," 205.

67. Evans, *Sexual Citizenship*, 5–6.

68. Solinger, *Beggars and Choosers*, 223–224.

69. Baer, *Biomedicine and Alternative Healing Systems in America*, 116; De Vries, *Making Midwives Legal*, 137.

70. Craven, "Making Our Voices Heard."

71. Martin et al., "Births," 16.

EPILOGUE: BEYOND CONSUMER RIGHTS

1. Jenkins, as cited in the Big Push for Midwives, "Father Knows Best Meets Big Brother Is Watching."

2. VABirthPAC Listserv message, Brynne Potter, 2008.

3. After the Governor's Work Group on Rural Obstetrical Care recommended removing physician supervision restrictions on CNMs to expand access to care in rural areas in 2004, legislation passed in 2005 supporting the establishment of CNM-run birth centers in Emporia and in the Northern Neck of Virginia, two "medically underserved" areas of the state. However, minimal funding for the venture was only approved in 2006. Thus, CNMs, led by project coordinator Jessica Jordan, continue their fundraising efforts privately to make the project a reality.

4. Commonwealth of Virginia, Department of Health Professions, "Public Information System."

5. Miller, "Public Argument and Legislative Debate in the Rhetorical Construction of Public Policy," 370.

6. Bourgeault, *Push!*, 280.

7. De Vries, *Making Midwives Legal*, 19.

8. Davis-Floyd, personal communication, April 21, 2010.

9. And despite the intensification of a "citizen as consumer" identity at the turn of the twenty-first century, it has a complicated history that spans much of the last hundred years. For an incisive, far more substantive look at this history, see Cohen, *A Consumer's Republic*.

10. Mukherjee, "'Ghetto Fabulous,'" 156. Roopali Mukherjee also argues persuasively that the adoption of the heavily racialized "bling aesthetic" in the context of the post-9/11 push toward patriotic consumerism has led to what she describes as the "death of civil rights," both for African Americans and ethnic immigrants.

11. Statement issued by Senator John D. Rockefeller IV, a Democrat from West Virginia. As cited in Stolberg, "'Public Option' in Health Plan May Be Dropped."

12. Patel, *Stuffed and Starved*, 312.

13. Ruzek, "Rethinking Feminist Ideologies and Actions," 307.

14. Midwives Alliance of North America, "MANA Position Statements."

15. Nelson, *Women of Color and the Reproductive Rights Movement*, 186.

16. Nelson, *Women of Color*; Silliman et al., *Undivided Rights*; Asian Communities for Reproductive Justice, "A New Vision for Advancing Our Movement for Reproductive Health, Reproductive Rights, and Reproductive Justice"; Smith, "Beyond Pro-Choice versus Pro-Life"; Solinger, *Pregnancy and Power*.

17. Solinger, *Pregnancy and Power*, 253.

Bibliography

Abu-Lughod, Lila. "Can There Be a Feminist Ethnography?" *Women and Performance: A Journal of Feminist Theory* 5(1), no. 9 (1990): 7–27.

———. *Veiled Sentiments: Honor and Poetry in a Bedouin Community.* Berkeley: University of California Press, 1986.

———. "Writing against Culture." In *Recapturing Anthropology: Working in the Present,* ed. Richard G. Fox, 137–162. Santa Fe, NM: School of American Research Press, 1991.

American College of Nurse-Midwives. "Certified Nurse-Midwives in Virginia," 2000. Available at www.midwife.org/prof/display.cfm?id=53, accessed July 29, 2002.

———. "The History of the American College of Nurse-Midwives." Available at www.midwife.org/about/history.cfm, accessed September 24, 2003.

———. "State by State Chart of Laws and Regulations That Need to Be Changed." Available at www.acnm.org/state_by_state_law.cfm, accessed July 8, 2009; last updated November 22, 2006.

———. "Certified Nurse-Midwives in Virginia," 2008. Available at www.midwife.org/siteFiles/legislative/Virginia_09.pdf, accessed April 10, 2010.

American College of Obstetricians and Gynecologists. "ACOG Statement on Home Births." Press release, February 6, 2008. Available at www.acog.org/from_home/publications/press_releases/nr02-06-08-2.cfm, accessed July 17, 2008.

American Medical Association. "Resolution 205, Subject: Home Deliveries." Available at www.ama-assn.org/ama/pub/category/18587.html, accessed July 17, 2008.

Amott, Teresa, and Julie Matthaei. *Race, Gender, and Work: A Multi-Cultural Economic History of Women in the United States.* Boston: South End Press, 1996.

Anzaldùa, Gloria, ed. *Borderlands/La Frontera: The New Mestiza.* San Francisco: Aunt Lute Books, 1987.

Arms, Suzanne. *Immaculate Deception: A New Look at Women and Childbirth in America*. New York: Bantam, 1975.

Asian Communities for Reproductive Justice. "A New Vision for Advancing Our Movement for Reproductive Health, Reproductive Rights, and Reproductive Justice," 2005. Available at www.reproductivejustice.org/reproductive.html, accessed August 7, 2009.

Baer, Hans. *Biomedicine and Alternative Healing Systems in America: Issues of Class, Race, Ethnicity, and Gender*. Madison: University of Wisconsin Press, 2001.

Baker, Lee. *From Savage to Negro: Anthropology and the Construction of Race, 1896–1954*. Berkeley: University of California Press, 1998.

Bambara, Toni Cade. *The Black Woman: An Anthology*. New York: Signet, 1970.

Baskervill, Bill. "House Panel Approves Apology for Eugenics: Forced Sterilizations Conducted until 1979." *The Associated Press*, January 30, 2001. Available at www.home.rica.net/airedale/Forced.htm, accessed December 5, 2007.

Baughman, Greer. "A Preliminary Report upon the Midwife Situation in Virginia." *Virginia Medical Monthly* 54 (1928): 748–751.

Baxandall, Rosalyn, Linda Gordon, and Susan Reverby. *America's Working Women*. New York: Random House, 1976.

Behar, Ruth, and Deborah A. Gordon. *Women Writing Culture*. Berkeley: University of California Press, 1995.

Bennett, Emily. "Midwife Work in Virginia." *Public Health Nurse* 17 (1925): 523–526.

Berino, Janna. "The History of Direct-Entry Midwifery in Florida." Speech delivered at the annual meetings of the Midwives Association of North America, Tampa, Florida, November 10, 2000.

The Big Push for Midwives. "Father Knows Best Meets Big Brother Is Watching: Physician Group Seeks to Outlaw Homebirth—Is Jail for Moms Next?" Press release, June 16, 2008. Available at www.thebigpushformidwives.org/pdf-bin/news.061608.pdf, accessed July 17, 2008.

———. "Number Two with a Bullet: Critical Women's Health Issues Neglected as Physician Group Yet Again Sets Its Sights on Midwives." Press release, September 1, 2008. Available at www.thebigpushformidwives.org/_ . . . /09-01-2008_PushNews_RELEASE_Number_Two_ With_a_Bullet.pdf, accessed July 23, 2009.

———. "The Push States." Available at www.thebigpushformidwives.org/index.cfm/fuseaction/home.stateStatus/index.htm, accessed April 16, 2010.

Biggs, Catherine L. "The Case of the Missing Midwives: A History of Midwifery in Ontario from 1795–1900." *Ontario History* 65(2) (1983): 21–25. Reprinted in *Delivering Motherhood: Maternal Ideologies and Practices in the 19th and 20th Centuries*, ed. Katherine Arnup, Andrée Levesque, and Ruth Roach Pierson, 20–36. London: Routledge, 1990.

Biggs, Lesley. "Rethinking the History of Midwifery in Canada." In *Reconceiving Midwifery*, ed. Ivy Lynn Bourgeault, Cecilia Benoit, and Robbie Davis-Floyd, 17–45. Montreal: McGill-Queen's University Press, 2004.

BirthCare and Women's Health. "BirthCare's History." Available at www.birthcare.org/history.htm, accessed April 10, 2010.

Block, Jennifer. *Pushed!: The Painful Truth about Childbirth and Modern Maternity Care*. Cambridge, MA: Da Capo Press, 2007.

Bobel, Chris. *The Paradox of Natural Mothering.* Philadelphia: Temple University Press, 2002.

Bookman, Ann, and Sandra Morgen. "Rethinking Women and Politics: An Introductory Essay." In *Women and the Politics of Empowerment,* ed. Ann Bookman and Sandra Morgen, 3–32. Philadelphia: Temple University Press, 1988.

———, eds. *Women and the Politics of Empowerment.* Philadelphia: Temple University Press. 1988.

Borst, Charlotte. *Catching Babies: The Professionalization of Childbirth, 1870–1920.* Cambridge, MA: Harvard University Press, 1995.

Boston Women's Health Collective. *Our Bodies, Ourselves: A Book By and For Women.* New York: Simon and Schuster, 1973.

Bourgeault, Ivy Lynn. *Push! The Struggle for Midwifery in Ontario.* Montreal: McGill-Queen's University Press, 2006.

Bourgeault, Ivy Lynn, Cecilia Benoit, and Robbie Davis-Floyd, eds. *Reconceiving Midwifery.* Montreal: McGill-Queen's University Press, 2004.

Briance, Prunella. *Natural Childbirth: Childbirth without Fear.* National Childbirth Trust Newsletter 2, March 1957.

Brown, Dennis, and Pamela A. Toussaint. *Mama's Little Baby: The Black Woman's Guide to Pregnancy, Childbirth and Baby's First Year.* New York: Plume, 1998.

Brown, Michael P. *Replacing Citizenship: AIDS Activism and Radical Democracy.* New York: Guildford Press, 1997.

Brown, S. S., ed. *Prenatal Care: Reaching Mothers, Reaching Infants.* Washington, DC: National Academy Press, 1988.

Caillagh, Cynthia L. Press release, May 5, 2000.

Carter, Patricia Cloyd. *Come Gently, Sweet Luciana.* Titusville, FL: Patricia Cloyd Carter, 1957.

Cassidy, Tina. *Birth: The Surprising History of How We Are Born.* New York: Grove Press, 2006.

Chafe, William Henry. *The American Woman: Her Changing Social, Economic, and Political Roles, 1920–1970.* New York: Oxford University Press, 1972.

Citizens for Midwifery. "What Is CfM?" Available at www.cfmidwifery.org/whatis/, accessed July 17, 2008.

Clifford, James, and George E. Marcus. *Writing Culture: The Poetics and Politics of Ethnography.* Berkeley: University of California Press, 1986.

Cobb, Ann Kuckelman. "Incorporation and Change: The Case of the Midwife in the United States." *Medical Anthropology* 5 (1981): 73–88.

Cohen, Lizabeth. *A Consumer's Republic: The Politics of Mass Consumption in Postwar America.* New York: Alfred A. Knopf, 2003.

Colen, Shellee. "'With Respect and Feelings': Voices of West Indian Childcare and Domestic Workers in New York City." In *All American Women: Lines That Divide, Ties That Bind,* ed. Johnnetta B Cole, 46–70. New York: Free Press, 1986.

Commonwealth of Virginia. *The Code of Virginia.* Available at www.leg1.state.va.us/000/src.htm, accessed March 10, 2003; last updated August 13, 2002.

———. "The Potential for the Expansion of the Practice of Nurse Midwives." House Joint Resolution 431, 1991.

———. "Study; direct-entry midwifery." Chief Patron Phillip A. Hamilton. Passed, March 22, 1999: House Joint Resolution 646. Available at www.leg1.state.va.us/cgi -bin/legp504.exe?ses=991&typ =bil&val=hj646, accessed December 5, 2007.

Commonwealth of Virginia, Department of Health, Center for Health Statistics. "Resident Live Home Births by Zip Code, Virginia." Unpublished MS, Virginia Center for Health Statistics, Richmond, 2000.

Commonwealth of Virginia, Department of Health Professions. "Public Information System: License Lookup," 2010. Available at www2.vipnet.org/dhp/cgi-bin/search _publicdb.cgi,accessed April 16, 2010.

Commonwealth of Virginia, Department of Health Professions and Virginia Health Planning Board, Task Force on the Study of Obstetric Access and Certified Nurse-Midwives. "The Potential for Expansion of the Practice of Nurse Midwives." House Document No. 12. Richmond: Commonwealth of Virginia, 1992.

Commonwealth of Virginia, Joint Commission on Health Care. "Midwifery Study Pursuant to HJR 646." House Document No. 76. Richmond: Commonwealth of Virginia, 2000.

———. "Summary of Public Comments: Midwifery Study (HJR 646)." Richmond: Commonwealth of Virginia, 2000.

Corea, Gena. *The Mother Machine.* New York: Harper and Row, 1985.

Cosslett, Tess. *Women Writing Childbirth: Modern Discourses of Childbirth.* Manchester: Manchester University Press, 1994.

Craven, Christa. "Claiming Respectable American Motherhood: Homebirth Mothers, Medical Officials, and the State." *Medical Anthropology Quarterly* 19, no. 2 (2005): 194–215.

———. "A 'Consumer's Right' to Choose a Midwife: Shifting Meanings for Reproductive Rights under Neoliberalism." *American Anthropologist* 109, no. 4 (2007): 701–712.

———. "Educated, Eliminated, Criminalized and Rediscovered: A History of Midwives in Virginia." Virginia Friends of Midwives, 2003. Formerly available at www .vfom.org. Updated version (2005) available at www.vabirthpac.org/historyofmid wifery.pdf, accessed April 10, 2010.

———. "'Every Breath Is Political, Every Woman's Life a Statement': Cross-Class Organizing for Midwifery in Virginia." In *Mainstreaming Midwives: The Politics of Change,* ed. Robbie Davis-Floyd and Christina Barbara Johnson, 311–346. New York: Routledge, 2006.

———. "Making Our Voices Heard: Highlighting Midwifery in Health Care Policy Debates." *Citizens for Midwifery News* 9, no. 2 (2004): 9–10.

Cross, Gary. *An All-Consuming Century: Why Commercialism Won in Modern America.* New York: Columbia University Press, 2000.

Cruikshank, Barbara. *The Will to Empower: Democratic Citizens and Other Subjects.* Ithaca, NY: Cornell University Press, 1999.

Davis, Dána-Ain. *Battered Black Women and Welfare Reform: Between a Rock and a Hard Place.* Albany: State University of New York Press, 2006.

———. "Knowledge in the Service of a Vision: Politically Engaged Anthropology." In *Engaged Observer: Anthropology, Advocacy, and Activism,* ed. Victoria Sanford and Asale Angel-Ajani, 228–238. New Brunswick, NJ: Rutgers University Press, 2006.

Davis-Floyd, Robbie. *Birth as an American Rite of Passage*. Berkeley: University of California Press, 1992.

———. "Consuming Childbirth: The Qualified Consumption of Midwifery Care." In *Consuming Motherhood*, ed. Janelle S. Taylor, Linda L. Layne, and Danielle F. Wozniak, 211–248. New Brunswick, NJ: Rutgers University Press, 2004.

———. "The Ups, Downs, and Interlinkages of Nurse- and Direct-Entry Midwifery: Status, Practice, and Education." Available at www.davis-floyd.com/art_index.html, accessed April 12, 2010. Originally printed in *Pathways to Becoming a Midwife: Getting an Education*, 4th ed. ed. Jan Tritten and Joel Southern, 67–118. Eugene, OR: Midwifery Today, 1998.

Davis-Floyd, Robbie, and Elizabeth Davis. "Intuition as Authoritative Knowledge in Midwifery and Home Birth." In *Childbirth and Authoritative Knowledge: Cross-cultural Perspectives*, ed. Robbie Davis-Floyd and Carolyn F. Sargent, 315–349. Berkeley: University of California Press, 1997.

Davis-Floyd, Robbie, and Joseph Dumit. "Cyborg Babies: Children of the Third Millenium [*sic*]." In *Cyborg Babies: From Techno-Sex to Techno-Tots*, ed. Robbie Davis-Floyd and Joseph Dumit, 1–18. New York: Routledge, 1998.

Davis-Floyd, Robbie, and Christina Barbara Johnson, eds. *Mainstreaming Midwifery. The Politics of Change*. New York: Routledge, 2006.

Davis-Floyd, Robbie, Stacey Leigh Pigg, and Sheila Cosminsky. "Introduction." Theme issue, "Daughters of Time: The Shifting Identities of Contemporary Midwives." *Medical Anthropology* 20, no. 2 (2001): 105–139.

Declerq, Eugene R., Lisa L. Paine, and Michael R. Winter. "Home Birth in the United States, 1989–1992: A Longitudinal Descriptive Report of National Birth Certificate Data." *Journal of Nurse-Midwifery* 40, no. 6 (1995): 474–482.

DeLee, Joseph B. "Progress toward Ideal Obstetrics." *American Journal of Obstetrics and Diseases of Women and Children* 73 (1916): 407–415.

Devitt, Neal. "The Statistical Case for Elimination of the Midwife: Fact versus Prejudice, 1890–1935 (Part 1)." *Women and Health* 4, no. 1 (Spring 1979): 81–96.

———. "The Statistical Case for Elimination of the Midwife: Fact versus Prejudice, 1890–1935 (Part 2)." *Women and Health* 4, no. 2 (Summer 1979): 169–186.

De Vries, Raymond, Cecilia Benoit, Edwin R. van Teijlingen, and Sirpa Wrede, eds. *Birth by Design: Pregnancy, Maternity Care, and Midwifery in North America and Europe*. New York: Routledge, 2001.

De Vries, Raymond G. *Making Midwives Legal: Childbirth, Medicine, and the Law*. 2nd ed. (orig. *Regulating Birth: Midwives, Medicine, and the Law*, 1986). Columbus: Ohio State University Press, 1996.

———. *Regulating Birth: Midwives, Medicine, and the Law*. Philadelphia: Temple University Press, 1986.

Dick-Read, Grantley. *Childbirth without Fear: The Principles and Practice of Natural Childbirth*. New York: Harper and Row, 1944[1933].

———. *No Time for Fear*. New York: Harper and Brothers, 1955.

Donegan, Jane B. *Women and Men Midwives: Medicine, Morality, and Misogyny in Early America*. Westport, CT: Greenwood Press, 1978.

Donnison, Jean. *Midwives and Medical Men: A History of Inter-Professional Rivalries and Women's Rights*. New York: Schocken Press, 1977.

Dougherty, Molly. "Southern Midwifery and Organized Health Care: Systems in Conflict." *Medical Anthropology* 6 (1982): 114–126.

Edwards, Diana S. "The Social Control of Illegitimacy through Adoption." *Human Organization* 58, no. 4 (1999): 387–396.

Edwards, Margot, and Mary Waldorf. *Reclaiming Birth: History and Heroines of American Childbirth Reform.* Trumansburg, NY: Crossing Press, 1984.

Ehrenreich, Barbara, and Deirdre English. *For Her Own Good: 150 Years of the Experts' Advice to Women.* New York: Anchor Books, 1978.

Evans, David T. *Sexual Citizenship: The Material Construction of Sexualities.* New York: Routledge, 1993.

Evans, Sara M. *Born for Liberty: A History of Women in America.* New York: Free Press, 1989.

Farmer, Paul. *Infections and Inequalities: The Modern Plagues.* Berkeley: University of California Press, 1999.

Fiedler, Deborah Cordero, and Robbie Davis-Floyd. "Midwifery as a Reproductive Right." In *Historical and Multicultural Encyclopedia of Women's Reproductive Rights in the United States,* ed. Judith A. Baer, 134–136. Westport, CT: Greenwood Press, 2001.

Fielding, Waldo, and Lois Benjamin. *The Childbirth Challenge: Commonsense versus "Natural" Methods.* New York: Viking, 1962.

Forster, Laura. "Welcome Home: Home Birth Creates Intimacy for Some, Controversy for Others." *Potomac News: Manassas Journal Messenger* (Prince Georges Region), November 26, 2000, A1, A4.

Foucault, Michel. "The Birth of Social Medicine." In *Power: Essential Works of Foucault 1954–1984,* vol. 3, ed. James D. Faubion, trans. Robert Hurley and others, 134–156. New York: New Press, 1994 [1974].

———. *Discipline and Punish: The Birth of the Prison.* New York: Vintage, 1979.

———. *The History of Sexuality, Volume 1: An Introduction.* New York: Vintage, 1980.

Fraser, Gertrude. *African American Midwifery in the South: Dialogues of Birth, Race and Memory.* Cambridge, MA: Harvard University Press, 1998.

———. "Afro-American Midwives, Biomedicine and the State: An Ethno-historical Account of Birth and Its Transformation in Rural Virginia." Ph.D. diss., Department of Anthropology, Johns Hopkins University, 1988.

———. "Modern Bodies, Modern Minds: Midwifery and Reproductive Change in an African American Community." In *Conceiving the New World Order: The Global Politics of Reproduction,* ed. Faye Ginsburg and Rayna Rapp, 42–58. Berkeley: University of California Press, 1995.

Freedman, Estelle. "Beyond the Waves: Rethinking the History of Feminism." In *Exploring Women's Studies: Looking Forward, Looking Back,* ed. Carol R. Berkin, Judith L. Pinch, and Carole S. Appel, 11–24. Upper Saddle River, NJ: Pearson Prentice Hall, 2006.

Gaskin, Ina May. *Spiritual Midwifery.* Summertown, TN: The Book Publishing Company, 1975.

Geertz, Clifford. "Thick Description: Toward an Interpretive Theory of Culture." In *The Interpretation of Cultures: Selected Essays,* 3–30. New York: Basic Books, 1973.

Gerheart, Melanie. "Joint Commission on Health Care to Study Lay Midwives and Obstetrical Education in Med Schools." *Virginia Section Review*, joint publication of the Virginia Obstetrical and Gynecological Society and the Virginia Section of the American College of Obstetricians and Gynecologists (Spring 1999): 2.

Gill, Leslie. *Teetering on the Rim: Global Restructuring, Daily Life, and the Armed Retreat of the Bolivian State*. New York: Columbia University Press, 2000.

Ginsburg, Faye. *Contested Lives: The Abortion Debate in an American Community*. Berkeley: University of California Press, 1989.

Ginsburg, Faye, and Rayna Rapp. "The Politics of Reproduction." *Annual Review of Anthropology* 20 (1991): 311–343.

Ginsburg, Faye, and Rayna Rapp, eds. *Conceiving the New World Order: The Global Politics of Reproduction*. Berkeley: University of California Press, 1995.

Glod, Maria, and Josh White. "Midwives Charged in Death of Va. Woman." *Washington Post*, January 21, 1999, B1.

Goldsmith, Judith. *Childbirth Wisdom: From the World's Oldest Societies*. Brookline, MA: East West Health Books, 1990.

Goode, Judith. "Let's Get Our Act Together: How Racial Discourses Disrupt Neighborhood Activism." In *The New Poverty Studies: The Ethnography of Power, Politics, and Impoverished People in the United States*, ed. Judith Goode and Jeff Maskovsky, 364–398. New York: New York University Press, 2001.

Goode, Judith, and Jeff Maskovsky, eds. *The New Poverty Studies: The Ethnography of Power, Politics, and Impoverished People in the United States*. New York: New York University Press, 2001.

Goodman, Deborah. "Trial Outcome." *Voices for Healthcare Rights Fund Newsletter*, July 2000.

Gordon, Deborah A. "Worlds of Consequences: Feminist Ethnography as Social Action." *Critique of Anthropology: A Journal for the Critical Reconstruction of Anthropology* 13, no. 4 (1993): 429–444.

Gordon, Linda. *The Moral Property of Women: A History of Birth Control Politics in America*. Urbana: University of Illinois Press, 2002.

———. *Pitied but Not Entitled: Single Mothers and the History of Welfare*. New York: Free Press, 1994.

———. "Voluntary Motherhood: The Beginnings of Feminist Birth Control Ideas in the United States." In *Women and Health in America*, ed. Judith Walzer Leavitt, 104–116. Madison: University of Wisconsin Press, 1999.

———. *Woman's Body, Woman's Right: A Social History of Birth Control in America*. New York: Penguin Books, 1974.

Governor's Work Group on Rural Obstetrical Care. "Executive Directive 2: Report of the Governor's Work Group on Rural Obstetrical Care," 2005. Available at www.vdh.virginia.gov/COMMISH/OBFinal_Report.pdf, accessed May 22, 2006.

Gray, Mary L. *Out in the Country: Youth, Media, and Queer Visibility in Rural America*. New York: New York University Press, 2009.

Greene, Julie. "Information Sheet: Peninsula Families for Natural Birth and Health Care-PenFam." Prepared for Virginia Midwifery Coalition, March 20, 1999, photocopy.

Grewal, Inderpal. *Transnational America: Feminisms, Diasporas, Neoliberalisms*. Durham, NC: Duke University Press, 2005.

Griesemer, Lynn M. *Unassisted Homebirth: An Act of Love*. Charleston, SC: Terra Publishing, 1998.

Haire, Doris. *The Cultural Warping of Childbirth: A Special Report*. Hillside, NJ: International Childbirth Education Association, 1972.

Hale, Charles. *Engaging Contradictions: Theory, Politics, and Methods of Activist Scholarship*. Berkeley: University of California Press, 2008.

Halfmoon, Hygeia. *Primal Mothering in a Modern World*. San Diego: Maul Brothers Publishing, 1998.

Hall, Jim. "The Decision, Cradle and Grave (Part 1)." *Free Lance-Star* (Fredericksburg, Virginia), January 26, 1998, A1, A4.

———. "Labor and Delivery, Cradle and Grave (Part 2)." *Free Lance-Star* (Fredericksburg, Virginia), January 27, 1998, A1, A4.

———. "The Descent, Cradle and Grave (Part 3)." *Free Lance-Star* (Fredericksburg, Virginia), January 28, 1998, A1, A10.

———. "The Midwife, Cradle and Grave (Part 4)." *Free Lance-Star* (Fredericksburg, Virginia), January 29, 1998, A1, A6.

———. "Death and Its Consequences, Cradle and Grave (Part 5)." *Free Lance-Star* (Fredericksburg, Virginia), January 30, 1998, A1, A14.

Haller, John S., Jr. *Medical Protestants: The Eclectics in American Medicine, 1825–1939*. Carbondale: Southern Illinois University Press, 1994.

Hamblet, Ellen. "Views of a Home Birth Advocate." *Virginia Capitol Connections Quarterly Magazine* 6, no. 3 (Summer 2000): 12–13.

Haraway, Donna. "Situated Knowledges: The Science Question in Feminism and the Privilege of Partial Perspective." *Feminist Studies* 14, no. 3 (1988): 575–599.

Hardin, E. R. "The Midwife Problem." *Southern Medical Journal* 18 (1925): 347–350.

Hardin, Peter. "'Documentary Genocide': Families' Surnames on Racial Hit List." *Richmond Times-Dispatch*, March 5, 2000, A1, A10, A12.

———. "Eugenics Affected Va. Law: Theory Advocated Social Engineering." *Richmond Times-Dispatch*, March 5, 2000, A11, A13.

Harrison, Faye. *Decolonizing Anthropology: Moving Further toward an Anthropology for Liberation*. 2nd ed. Arlington, VA: Association of Black Anthropologists and American Anthropological Association, 1991.

———. "Feminist Methodology as a Tool for Ethnographic Inquiry on Globalization." In *The Gender of Globalization: Women Navigating Cultural and Economic Marginalities*, ed. Nandini Gunewardena and Ann Kingsolver, 23–31. Santa Fe, NM: School for Advanced Research Press, 2007.

———. "Gender, Sexuality and Health in a Turn-of-the-Century 'Black Metropolis.'" *Medical Anthropology Quarterly* 11, no. 4 (1997): 448–453.

Harvey, David. *A Brief History of Neoliberalism*. New York: Oxford University Press, 2005.

Hatch, Jenny. Online book review of Lynn M. Griesemer's *Unassisted Homebirth: An Act of Love* (1998). Available at www.unassistedhomebirth.com/bookreviews.html, accessed October 16, 2009.

Hazell, Lester Dessez. *Birth Goes Home: An Ethnographic and Attitudinal Study of 300 Couples Electing Home Birth in the San Francisco Bay Area.* Seattle, WA: Catalyst Publishing, 1974.

Heiligman, D. "The Birthing Center Experience." *Parent's Magazine* 65, no. 10 (October 1990): 70.

Heneghan, Georgia. "They've Come a Long Way, Baby, Midwives: A Tradition Reborn (Part 1)." *Free Lance-Star* (Fredericksburg, Virginia), March 14, 1990, 33–35.

Heyser, Holly. "Midwifery Expansion Fails as Proposal from Health Panel." *Virginian-Pilot* (Norfolk, Virginia), January 9, 2000, B2.

Hoebel, E. Adamson, and Thomas Weaver. *Anthropology and the Human Experience.* 5th ed. New York: McGraw-Hill, 1979.

Holland, Dorothy, Donald M. Nonini, Catherine Lutz, Lesley Bartlett, Marla Frederick-McGlathery, Thaddeus C. Guldbrandsen, and Enrique G. Murillo Jr. *Local Democracy under Siege: Activism, Public Interests and Private Politics.* New York: New York University Press, 2007.

Holmes, Linda Janet. "African American Midwives in the South." In *The American Way of Birth*, ed. Pamela Eakins, 273–291. Philadelphia: Temple University Press, 1986.

Horton, J. A. *The Women's Health Data Book: A Profile of Women's Health in the United States.* 2nd ed. Washington, DC: Jacobs Institute for Women's Health, 1995.

Hughes, Martha, and Trinlie Wood. "Information Sheet for Commonwealth Midwives Alliance." Prepared for Virginia Midwifery Coalition, March 20, 1999, photocopy.

Hyatt, Susan Brin. "From Citizen to Volunteer: Neoliberal Governance and the Erasure of Poverty." In *The New Poverty Studies: The Ethnography of Power, Politics, and Impoverished People in the United States*, ed. Judith Goode and Jeff Maskovsky, 201–235. New York: New York University Press, 2001.

———. "Poverty and the Medicalisation of Motherhood." In *Sex, Gender and Health*, ed. Teresa M. Pollard and Susan Brin Hyatt, 94–117. New York: Cambridge University Press, 1999.

Inhorn, Marcia C., and Frank Van Balen. *Infertility around the Globe: New Thinking on Childlessness, Gender, and Reproductive Technologies.* Berkeley: University of California Press, 2002.

Irving, Frederick. *Safe Deliverance.* Boston: Houghton Mifflin Company, 1942.

Jenkins, Gwynne. "Burning Bridges: Policy, Practice, and the Destruction of Midwifery in Rural Costa Rica," *Social Science & Medicine* 56, no. 9 (2003): 1893–1909.

Jolly, Margaret, and Kalpana Ram. *Borders of Being: Citizenship, Fertility, and Sexuality in Asia and the Pacific.* Ann Arbor: University of Michigan Press, 2001.

Jones, Gordon. "Will There Be a Place for Nurse Midwives?" *Virginia Medical Monthly* 43 (1966): 173–175.

Jordan, Brigitte. "Authoritative Knowledge and Its Construction." In *Childbirth and Authoritative Knowledge: Cross-cultural Perspectives*, ed. Robbie Davis-Floyd and Carolyn Sargent, 55–79. Berkeley: University of California Press, 1997.

———. *Birth in Four Cultures: A Cross-cultural Investigation of Childbirth in Yucatan, Holland, Sweden, and the United States.* Prospect Heights, IL: Waveland Press, 1978.

Kahn, Robbie Pfeufer. *Bearing Meaning: The Language of Birth*. Urbana: University of Illinois Press, 1995.

Kaplan, Laura. *The Story of Jane: The Legendary Underground Feminist Abortion Service*. New York: Pantheon Books, 1995.

Karmel, Marjorie. *Thank You, Dr. Lamaze: A Mother's Experiences in Painless Childbirth*. Philadelphia: Lippincott, 1959.

Katz, Barbara. "Childbirth and the Law." *Colorado Medicine* 77, no. 2 (1980): 64–68.

Kessler-Harris, Alice. *In Pursuit of Equity: Women, Men, and the Quest for Economic Citizenship in 20th-Century America*. Oxford: Oxford University Press, 2001.

Kingfisher, Catherine, and Jeff Maskovsky. "Introduction: The Limits of Neoliberalism." *Critique of Anthropology* 28. no. 2 (2008): 115–126.

Kitzinger, Jenny. "Strategy of the Early Childbirth Movement: A Case Study of the National Childbirth Trust." In *The Politics of Maternity Care*, ed. Jo Garcia, Robert Kilpatrick, and Martin Richards, 154–168. London: Oxford University Press, 1990.

Kitzinger, Sheila. *Birth at Home*. Oxford: Oxford University Press, 1979.

———. *The Experience of Childbirth*. New York: Taplinger, 1972[1962].

———, ed. *Giving Birth: How It Really Feels* [originally published as *Giving Birth: The Parents' Emotions in Childbirth*, 1961]. London: Victor Gollancz, 1987.

———. *Women as Mothers: How They See Themselves in Different Cultures*. New York: Random House, 1978.

Klassen, Pamela E. *Blessed Events: Religion and Homebirth in America*. Princeton, NJ: Princeton University Press, 2001.

———. "Mothers between God and Mammon: Feminist Interpretations of Childbirth." In *Consuming Motherhood*, ed. Janelle S. Taylor, Linda L. Layne, and Danielle F. Wozniak, 249–268. New Brunswick, NJ: Rutgers University Press, 2004.

Klaus, Marshall, John Kennell, and Phyllis Klaus. *The Doula Book*. 2nd ed. Cambridge, MA: Perseus, 2002[1993].

Krauss, Celene. "Women of Color on the Front Line." In *Unequal Protection: Environmental Justice and Communities of Color*, ed. Robert D. Bullard, 256–271. San Francisco: Sierra Club Books, 1994.

Krishnamurthy, Kiran. "Midwife Expected to Enter Guilty Plea." *Richmond Times-Dispatch*, May 5, 2000, B4.

———. "Unlicensed Midwives Get Jail Sentences." *Richmond Times-Dispatch*, May 6, 2000, A1.

Ladd-Taylor, Molly. "'Grannies' and 'Spinsters': Midwife Education under the Sheppard-Towner Act." *Journal of Social History* 22 (1988): 255–275.

Lamaze, Ferdinand. *Painless Childbirth: The Lamaze Method*. New York: Pocket Books, 1956.

Lamphere, Louise, Patricia Zavella, and Felipe Gonzales, with Peter B. Evans. *Sunbelt Working Mothers: Reconciling Family and Factory*. Ithaca, NY: Cornell University Press, 1993.

Langston, A. "Diagnosis and Normal Delivery." *Virginia Medical Monthly* 56 (1929): 379–382.

Lapp, Hannah. "The Home-Birth Controversy." *The Freeman* (a publication of the Foundation for Economic Education) 42, no. 6 (1992). Available at www.fee.org/news.php?nid=2588, accessed December 5, 2007.

Lassiter, Luke Eric. *The Chicago Guide to Collaborative Ethnography*. Chicago: University of Chicago Press, 2005.

Lay, Mary M. "The Legal Status of Direct-Entry Midwives in the United States: Balancing Tradition with Modern Medicine." In *Body Talk: Rhetoric, Technology, Reproduction*, ed. Mary M. Lay, Laura J. Gurak, Clare Gravon, and Cynthia Myntti, 226–243. Madison: University of Wisconsin Press, 2000.

———. *The Rhetoric of Midwifery: Gender, Knowledge, and Power*. New Brunswick, NJ: Rutgers University Press, 2000.

Layne, Linda. *Motherhood Lost: A Feminist Account of Pregnancy Loss in America*. New York: Routledge, 2003.

Lazarus, Ellen. "What Do Women Want? Issues of Choice, Control, and Class in American Pregnancy and Childbirth." In *Childbirth and Authoritative Knowledge: Cross-cultural Perspectives*, ed. Robbie Davis-Floyd and Carolyn Sargent, 132–158. Berkeley: University of California Press, 1997.

Leavitt, Judith Walzer. *Brought to Bed: Childbearing in America, 1750–1950*. New York: Oxford University Press, 1986.

———. "'Science' Enters the Birthing Room: Obstetrics in America since the Eighteenth Century." *Journal of American History* 70, no. 2 (1983): 281 304.

Lee, Valerie. *Granny Midwives and Black Women Writers: Double-Dutched Readings*. New York: Routledge, 1996.

Lemons, Stanley J. *The Woman Citizen: Social Feminism in the 1920s*. Urbana: University of Illinois Press, 1973.

Leupp, Constance, and Burton J. Hendrick. "Twilight Sleep in America." *McClure's Magazine* 44 (1915): 172–173.

Litoff, Judy Barrett, ed. *The American Midwifery Debate: A Sourcebook on Its Origins*. New York: Greenwood Press, 1986.

———. *American Midwives: 1860 to the Present*. Westport, CT: Greenwood Press, 1978.

Lock, Margaret, and Patricia Kaufert. *Pragmatic Women and Body Politics*. Cambridge: Cambridge University Press, 1998.

Lombardo, Paul. "Eugenic Sterilization in Virginia: Aubrey Strode and the Case of Buck V. Bell." Ph.D. diss., School of Education, University of Virginia, 1982.

Lopez, Iris. "Agency and Constraint: Sterilization and Reproductive Freedom among Puerto Rican Women in New York City." In *Situated Lives: Gender and Culture in Everyday Life*, ed. Louise Lamphere, Helena Ragoné, and Patricia Zavella, 157–171. New York: Routledge, 1997.

Lorde, Audre. *Zami: A New Spelling of My Name*. Watertown, MA: Persephone Press, 1982.

Luker, Kristin. *Abortion and the Politics of Motherhood*. Berkeley: University of California Press, 1984.

Lyon-Callo, Vincent. *Inequality, Poverty, and Neoliberal Governance: Activist Ethnography in the Homeless Sheltering Industry*. Peterborough, Ontario: Broadview Press, 2004.

Mabbott, J. "The Regulation of Midwives in New York." *American Journal of Obstetrics* 55 (1907): 516–527.

Macari, Marcie. *She Births: A Modern Woman's Guidebook for an Ancient Rite of Passage*. West Coshohocken, PA: Infinity Publishing, 2006.

MacDonald, Margaret. *At Work in the Field of Birth: Midwifery Narratives of Nature, Tradition, and Home*. Nashville, TN: Vanderbilt University Press, 2007.

———. "Postmodern Negotiations with Medical Technology: The Role of Midwifery Clients in the New Midwifery in Canada." *Medical Anthropology* 20 (2001): 245–276.

———. "Tradition as a Political Symbol in the New Midwifery in Canada." In *Reconceiving Midwifery*, ed. Ivy Lynn Bourgeault, Cecilia Benoit, and Robbie Davis-Floyd, 46–66. Montreal: McGill-Queen's University Press, 2004.

MacDonald, Margaret, and Ivy Lynn Bourgeault. "The Politics of Representation: Doing and Writing 'Interested' Research on Midwifery." *Resources for Feminist Research/ Documentation sur la Recherche Féministe* 28, nos. 1–2 (2000): 151–168.

MAMA Campaign. "The Midwives and Mothers in Action (MAMA) Campaign Is Launched!" Available at www.mamacampaign.org, accessed July 7, 2009.

Mander, Rosemary, and Valerie Flemming. *Failure to Progress: The Contraction of the Midwifery Profession*. New York: Routledge, 2002.

Mander, Rosemary, and Lindsay Reid. "Midwifery Power." In *Failure to Progress: The Contraction of the Midwifery Profession*, ed. Rosemary Mander and Valerie Flemming, 1–19. New York: Routledge, 2002.

Marable, Manning, and Leith Mullings, eds. *Let Nobody Turn Us Around: Voices of Resistance, Reform, and Renewal: An African American Anthology*. Lanham, MD: Rowan and Littlefield, 2000.

Marcus, George. "Ethnography in/of the World System: The Emergence of Multi-Sited Ethnography." *Annual Review of Anthropology* 24 (1995): 95–117.

Martin, Emily. *The Woman in the Body*. Boston: Beacon Press, 1987.

Martin, Joyce A., Brady E. Hamilton, Paul D. Sutton, Stephanie J. Ventura, Fay Menacker, Sharon Kirmeyer, and T.J. Mathews. "Births: Final Data for 2006." United States of America, Center for Disease Control, National Center for Health Statistics, National Vital Statistics Report 57, no. 7 (2009). Hyattsville, MD: National Center for Health Statistics. Available at www.cdc.gov/Nchs/fastats/births.htm, accessed April 18, 2010.

Maskovsky, Jeff. "'Managing' the Poor: Neoliberalism, Medicaid HMOs, and the Triumph of Consumerism among the Poor." *Medical Anthropology* 19, no. 2 (2000): 127–172.

Mathews, Holly F. "Killing the Medical Self-Help Tradition among African Americans: The Case of Lay Midwifery in North Carolina, 1912–1983." In *African Americans in the South: Issues of Race, Class, and Gender*, ed. Hans Baer and Yvonne Jones, 60–78. Athens: University of Georgia Press, 1992.

Mathews, Joan J., and Kathleen Zadak. "The Alternative Birth Movement in the United States: History and Current Status." *Women and Health* 17, no. 1 (1991): 39–56.

Matthews, Jean V. *The Rise of the New Woman: The Women's Movement in America, 1875–1930*. Chicago: Ivan R. Dee, 2003.

McCarthy, John D., and Mayer N. Zald. "Resource Mobilization and Social Movements: A Partial Theory." *American Journal of Sociology* 82, no. 6 (1977): 1212–1241.

McGregor, R. R. *Herbal Birth Control: A Brief History with Ancient and Modern Herbal Recipes*. Weatherford, OK: Cloud Chief Publishing, 1993.

McNurlin, C. A. "Giving Birth: New Options for Expectant Parents." *Better Homes and Gardens* 65 (November 1986): 97–99.

Mead, Margaret. *Blackberry Winter: My Early Years*. New York: Morrow, 1972.

Mehl, L. "Statistical Outcomes of Homebirth in the U.S.: Current Status." In *Safe Alternatives in Childbirth*, ed. David Stewart and Lee Stewart, 127–141. Chapel Hill, NC: National Association of Parents and Professionals for Safe Alternatives in Childbirth, 1976.

Michaelson, Karen. "Childbirth in America: A Brief History and Contemporary Issues." In *Childbirth in America: Anthropological Perspectives*, ed. Karen Michaelson, 1–32. South Hadley, MA: Bergin and Garvey, 1988.

Michie, Helena, and Naomi R. Cahn. "Unnatural Births: Cesarean Sections in the Discourse of the 'Natural Childbirth' Movement." In *Gender and Health: An International Perspective*, ed. Carolyn F. Sargent and Caroline Brettell, 44–56. Upper Saddle River, NJ: Prentice Hall, 1996.

Midwives Alliance of North America. "MANA Position Statements." Adopted by MANA Board, May 1994. Available at www.mana.org/positions.html, accessed July 16, 2008.

———. "Mission Statement." Available at www.mana.org, accessed May 22, 2003; last updated April 17, 2003.

Miller, M. Linda. "Public Argument and Legislative Debate in the Rhetorical Construction of Public Policy: The Case of Florida Midwifery Legislation." *The Quarterly Journal of Speech* 85, no. 4 (1999): 361–379.

Mohanty, Chandra Talpade. *Feminism without Borders: Decolonizing Theory, Practicing Solidarity*. Durham, NC: Duke University Press, 2003.

Mohr, James. *Abortion in America: The Origins and Evolution of National Policy*. New York: Oxford University Press, 1978.

Mongeau, Beatrice. "The 'Granny' Midwife: Changing Roles and Functions of a Folk Practitioner." *American Journal of Sociology* 66 (1961): 497–505.

Morgan, Lynn, and Elizabeth Roberts. "Rights and Reproduction in Latin America." *Anthropology News* (March 2009): 12, 16.

Morgen, Sandra. *Into Our Own Hands: The Women's Health Movement in the United States, 1969–1990*. New Brunswick, NJ: Rutgers University Press, 2002.

———. "'It's the Whole Power of the City against Us!': The Development of Political Consciousness in a Women's Health Care Coalition." In *Women and the Politics of Empowerment*, ed. Ann Bookman and Sandra Morgen, 97–115. Philadelphia: Temple University Press, 1988.

MotherBirth. "Frequently Asked Questions about Doulas." Available at www.motherbirth.com/Doula%20FAQ.htm, accessed July 21, 2009.

Mukherjee, Roopali. "'Ghetto Fabulous' in the Imperial United States: Black Consumption and the 'Death of Civil Rights.'" In *Rethinking America: The Imperial Homeland in the 21st Century*, ed. Jeff Maskovsky and Ida Susser, 148–163. Boulder, CO: Paradigm, 2009.

Mullings, Leith. "Households Headed by Women: The Politics of Race, Class, and Gender." In *Conceiving the New World Order: The Global Politics of Reproduction*, ed. Faye Ginsburg and Rayna Rapp, 120–139. Berkeley: University of California Press, 1995.

———. "Inequality and African American Health Status: Policies and Prospects." In *Race: 20th Century Dilemmas, 21st Century Prognoses*, ed. Winston A. Van Horne, 154–182. Madison: University of Wisconsin Press, 1989.

———. *On Our Own Terms: Race, Class, and Gender in the Lives of African American Women*. New York: Routledge, 1997.

Murray, William L. "Direct Entry Midwifery Study by Senior Health Policy Analyst for the Joint Commission on Health Care." PowerPoint presentation to the Commonwealth of Virginia, General Assembly, Joint Commission on Health Care, Midwifery Subcommittee. Richmond, Virginia, July 27, 1999.

———. "Staff Follow-up from Last Meeting by Senior Health Policy Analyst for the Joint Commission on Health Care." Presentation to the Commonwealth of Virginia, General Assembly, Joint Commission on Health Care, Midwifery Subcommittee. Richmond, Virginia, August 6, 1999.

Mwaria, Cheryl. "Diversity in the Context of Health and Illness." In *Cultural Diversity in the United States*, ed. Ida Susser and Thomas Patterson, 57–75. Malden, MA: Blackwood, 2001.

Nader, Ralph. "Introduction." In *The Monopoly Makers: Ralph Nader's Study Group Report on Regulation and Competition*, ed. Mark J. Green, ix–xv. New York: Grossman, 1973.

Naples, Nancy. *Grassroots Warriors: Activist Mothering, Community Work, and the War on Poverty*. New York: Routledge, 1998.

National Organization for Women. "1999 NOW Conference Resolutions, Expansion of Reproductive Freedom to Include the Midwifery Model of Care." Available at www.now.org/nnt/fall-99/resolutions.html#midwifery, accessed December 5, 2007.

Nelson, Jennifer. *Women of Color and the Reproductive Rights Movement*. New York: New York University Press, 2003.

Nelson, Margaret. "Working-Class Women, Middle-Class Women, and Models of Childbirth." *Social Problems* 30, no. 3 (1983): 284–297.

Nestel, Sheryl. "The Boundaries of Professional Belonging: How Race Has Shaped the Re-Emergence of Midwifery in Ontario." In *Reconceiving Midwifery*, ed. Ivy Lynn Bourgeault, Cecilia Benoit, and Robbie Davis-Floyd, 287–305. Montreal: McGill-Queen's University Press, 2004.

———. *Obstructed Labour: Race and Gender in the Re-Emergence of Midwifery*. Vancouver: University of British Columbia Press, 2006.

———. "'Other Mothers': Race and Representation in Natural Childbirth Discourse." *Resources for Feminist Research/Documentation sur la Recherche Féministe* 23, no. 4 (1995): 5–19.

Nestle, Joan. *A Restricted Country*. Ithaca, NY: Firebrand Books, 1987.

Neuberger, Christine. "Officials Explain Charges against Two Midwives." *Richmond Times-Dispatch*, January 29, 1999, B1.

———. "Traditional Midwife Extols Value, Rewards She Discovered." *Richmond Times-Dispatch*, Area/State, March 1, 1999, A1.

Norris, Lynn. "Birthrites: Midwife Brings Art to Life." *Riverviews: Northcumberland Echo and Westmoreland and Northern Neck News* (July 1995): 72, 74.

North American Registry of Midwives. "CPM Brochure Text," 1996. Available at www.narm.org/brochurecontent.htm, accessed July 30, 2008; last updated May 1996.

———. "North American Registry of Midwives Mission Statement," 2008. Available at www.narm.org/htb.htm#mission, accessed July 8, 2009; last updated January 28, 2008.

Numbers, Ronald L. "Do-It-Yourself the Sectarian Way." In *Sickness and Health in America: Readings in the History of Medicine and Public Health*, 1st ed., ed. Judith Walzer Leavitt and Ronald L., 87–96 Madison: University of Wisconsin Press, 1978.

Oakley, Ann. *Women Confined: Toward a Sociology of Childbirth*. New York: Schocken Books, 1980.

Oakley, Ann, and Susanne Houd. *Helpers in Childbirth: Midwifery Today*. New York: Hemisphere, 1990.

Ordover, Nancy. *American Eugenics: Race, Queer Anatomy, and the Science of Nationalism*. Minneapolis: University of Minnesota Press, 2003.

Parker, Jennifer D. "Ethnic Differences in Midwife-Attended US Births." *American Journal of Public Health* 84, no. 7 (July 1994): 1139–1141.

Parnall, Christopher. "Nursing and the Health of the Future." *Public Health Nursing* 13 (1921): 573–578.

Parsons, Ethel. "Child Hygiene and Public Health Nursing." *Public Health Nursing* 13 (1921): 285–287.

Pasveer, Bernike, and Madeleine Akrich. "Obstetrical Trajectories: On Training Women/Bodies for (Home) Birth." In *Birth by Design: Pregnancy, Maternity Care, and Midwifery in North America and Europe*, ed. Raymond De Vries, Cecilia Benoit, Edwin R. van Teijlingen, and Sirpa Wrede, 229–242. New York: Routledge, 2001.

Patel, Raj. *Stuffed and Starved: The Hidden Battle for the World Food System*. Brooklyn, NY: Melville House, 2007.

Pegram, Cynthia T. "Unlicensed Midwives Can't Practice Legally under Virginia Statute." *The News & Advance* (Lynchburg, Virginia), August 18, 1996, B1, B5.

Petchesky, Rosalind Pollack. *Abortion and Woman's Choice: The State, Sexuality, and Reproductive Freedom*. New York: Longman, 1984.

Plecker, William A. "Surnames by Counties and Cities, Virginia Families Striving to Pass as 'Indian' and/or White." Letter to Local Registrars, Physicians, Health Officers, Nurses, School Superintendents and Clerks of the Courts, January 1943. Available at www.vcdh.virginia.edu/lewisandclark/encounter/projects/monacans/ Contemporary_Monacans/letter.html, accessed July 17, 2003.

———. "Virginia Makes Efforts to Solve Midwife Problem." *The Nation's Health* 8, no. 12 (1925): 809–811.

Rapp, Rayna. *Testing Women, Testing the Fetus: The Social Impact of Amniocentesis in America*. New York: Routledge, 1999.

Reid, Margaret. "Sisterhood and Professionalization: A Case Study of the American Lay Midwife." In *Women as Healers: Cross-cultural Perspectives*, ed. Carol Shepherd McClain, 219–238. New Brunswick, NJ: Rutgers University Press, 1995.

Rich, Adrienne. *Of Woman Born: Motherhood as Experience and Institution*. New York: Norton, 1976.

Riddle, John M. *Contraception and Abortion from the Ancient World to the Renaissance*. Cambridge, MA: Harvard University Press, 1992.

Robinson, Caroline Hadley. *Seventy Birth Control Clinics*. Baltimore, MD: Williams and Wilkins, 1930.

Robnett, Belinda. "African-American Women in the Civil Rights Movement, 1954–1965: Gender, Leadership, and Micromobilization." *American Journal of Sociology* 101, no. 6 (May 1996): 1661–1693.

Romalis, Shelley. "An Overview." In *Childbirth: Alternatives to Medical Control*, ed. Shelley Romalis, 3–33. Austin: University of Texas Press, 1981.

Romalis, Shelley, ed. *Childbirth: Alternatives to Medical Control*. Austin: University of Texas Press, 1981.

Rooks, Judith Pence. *Midwifery and Childbirth in America*. Philadelphia: Temple University Press, 1997.

Ross, Loretta J. "African-American Women and Abortion: 1800–1970." In *Theorizing Black Feminisms: The Visionary Pragmatism of Black Women*, ed. Stanlie M. James and Abena P. A. Busia, 141–159. London: Routledge, 1993.

Roth, Rachel. "Justice Denied: Violations of Women's Reproductive Rights in the United States Prison System," *Pro-Choice Forum*, September 2004. Available at www.prochoiceforum.org.uk/psy_ocr10.php, accessed July 31, 2009.

———. *Making Women Pay: The Hidden Costs of Fetal Rights*. Ithaca, NY: Cornell University Press, 2000.

Rothman, Barbara Katz. "Awake and Aware, or False Consciousness: The Co-optation of Childbirth Reform in America." In *Childbirth: Alternatives to Medical Control*, ed. Shelly Romalis, 150–180. Austin: University of Texas Press, 1981.

———. "Caught in the Current." In *Consuming Motherhood*, ed. Janelle S. Taylor, Linda L. Layne, and Danielle F. Wozniak, 279–288. New Brunswick, NJ: Rutgers University Press, 2004.

———. *In Labor: Women and Power in the Birthplace*. New York: W.W. Norton & Company, 1982.

———. *In Labor: Women and Power in the Birthplace*, 2nd ed. New York: W.W. Norton & Company, 1991.

———. *Recreating Motherhood: Ideology and Technology in Patriarchal Society*. New York: W.W. Norton & Company, 1989.

Rothman, Sheila M. *Women's Proper Place: A History of Changing Ideals and Practices, 1870 to the Present*. New York: Basic Books, 1978.

Rothstein, William G. *American Physicians in the Nineteenth Century: From Sects to Science*. Baltimore, MD: Johns Hopkins University Press, 1972.

Ruzek, Sheryl Burt. "Rethinking Feminist Ideologies and Actions: Thoughts on the Past and Future of Health Reform." In *Revisioning Women, Health, and Healing: Feminist, Cultural, and Technoscience Perspectives*, ed. Adele E. Clarke and Virginia L. Olesen, 303–323. New York: Routledge, 1999.

———. *The Women's Health Movement: Feminist Alternatives to Medical Control*. New York: Praeger, 1978.

Ruzek, Sheryl Burt, Virginia L. Olesen, and Adele E. Clarke, eds. *Women's Health: Complexities and Differences*. Columbus: Ohio University Press, 1997.

Sacks, Karen. *Caring by the Hour: Women, Work, and Organizing at Duke Medical Center*. Urbana: University of Illinois Press, 1988.

Sandel, Michael J. *Democracy's Discontent: America in Search of a Public Philosophy.* Cambridge, MA: Belknap Press of Harvard University Press, 1996.

Sandelowski, Margarete. *Pain, Pleasure, and American Childbirth: From the Twilight Sleep to the Read Method, 1914–1960.* Westport, CT: Greenwood Press, 1984.

Sanford, Victoria. "Introduction." In *Engaged Observer: Anthropology, Advocacy, and Activism,* ed. Victoria Sanford and Asale Angel-Ajani, 1–15. New Brunswick, NJ: Rutgers University Press, 2006.

Sanford, Victoria, and Asale Angel-Ajani. *Engaged Observer: Anthropology, Advocacy, and Activism.* New Brunswick, NJ: Rutgers University Press, 2006.

Sawicki, Jana. *Disciplining Foucault: Feminism, Power, and the Body.* New York: Routledge, 1991.

Schlenzka, Peter. "Safety of Alternative Approaches to Childbirth." Ph.D. diss., Department of Sociology, Stanford University, 1999.

Schlinger, Hilary. *Circle of Midwives: Organized Midwifery in North America.* LaFayette, NY: Schlinger, 1992.

Schmalhauser, Sam. "The Twilight Sleep for Women." *International Socialist Review* 15 (1914): 234–235.

Schoen, Johanna. "Reconceiving Abortion: Medical Practice, Women's Access, and Feminist Politics before and after *Roe v. Wade.*" *Feminist Studies* 26, no. 2 (2000): 349–376.

Schor, Juliet. *The Overspent American: Upscaling, Downshifting, and the New Consumer.* New York: Basic Books, 1998.

Scully, Diana. *Men Who Control Women's Health: The Miseducation of Obstetrician-Gynecologists.* Boston: Houghton-Mifflin, 1980.

Shanley, Laura, and Mairi Breen-Rothman. "Freebirth Movement." *Washington Post,* transcript of online discussion from July 31, 2007. Available at www.washingtonpost.com/wp-dyn/content/discussion/2007/07/27/DI2007072701583.html, accessed July 20, 2009.

Shanley, Laura Kaplan. *Unassisted Childbirth.* Westport, CT: Bergin & Garvey, 1994.

Shaw, Nancy Stoller. *Forced Labor: Maternity Care in the United States.* New York: Pergamon Press, 1974.

Shryock, Richard Harrison. *Medicine in America: Historical Essays.* Baltimore, MD: Johns Hopkins University Press, 1966.

Silliman, Jael, Marlene Gerber Fried, Loretta Ross, and Elena R. Gutiérrez. *Undivided Rights: Women of Color Organize for Reproductive Justice.* Cambridge, MA: South End Press, 2004.

Simonds, Wendy, Barbara Katz Rothman, and Bari Meltzer Norman. *Laboring On: Birth in Transition in the United States.* New York: Routledge, 2007.

Skocpol, Theda. *Protecting Soldiers and Mothers: The Political Origins of Social Policy in the United States.* Cambridge, MA: Harvard University Press, 1992.

Smith, Andrea. "Beyond Pro-Choice versus Pro-Life: Women of Color and Reproductive Justice." *NWSA Journal* 17, no. 1 (2005): 119–140.

Smith, Claudine Curry, and Mildred Baker Roberson. *Memories of a Black Lay Midwife from Northern Neck Virginia.* Lisle, IL: Tucker Publications, 1994.

————. *My Bag Was Always Packed: The Life and Times of a Virginia Midwife.* Bloomington, IN: First Books, 2003.

Smith, Margaret Charles, and Linda Janet Holmes. *Listen to Me Good: The Life Story of an Alabama Midwife.* Columbus: Ohio State University Press, 1996.

Solinger, Rickie. *Beggars and Choosers: How the Politics of Choice Shapes Adoption, Abortion, and Welfare.* New York: Hill and Wang, 2001.

————. *Pregnancy and Power: A Short History of Reproductive Politics in America.* New York: Routledge, 2005.

Sousa, Marion. *Childbirth at Home.* New York: Bantam, 1976.

Stacey, Judith. "Can There Be a Feminist Ethnography?" *Women's Studies International Forum* 11, no. 1 (1988): 21–27.

Stern, Howard. "A Public Health Perspective on Midwifery by the Director of the Office of Family Health Services, Virginia Department of Health." A PowerPoint presentation to the Commonwealth of Virginia, General Assembly, Joint Commission on Health Care. Richmond, Virginia, August 10, 1999.

Stevens, Rosemary. *In Sickness and in Wealth: American Hospitals in the Twentieth Century.* New York: Basic Books, 1986.

Stewart, David. "Homebirths—A Modern Trend—Is It Progress?" In *Safe Alternatives in Childbirth,* ed. David Stewart and Lee Stewart, 5–11. Chapel Hill, NC: National Association of Parents and Professionals for Safe Alternatives in Childbirth, 1976.

Stillman, Carla G. "Painless Childbirth." *New York Call* (July 12, 1914): 15.

Stolberg, Sheryl Gay. "'Public Option' in Health Plan May Be Dropped." *New York Times,* August 17, 2009, A1.

Strobel, Jennifer. "Going Back to the Roots, Midwives: A Tradition Reborn (Part 2)." *Free Lance-Star* (Fredericksburg, Virginia), March 15, 1990, 27–28.

Sullivan, Deborah A., and Rose Weitz. *Labor Pains: Modern Midwives and Home Birth.* New Haven, CT: Yale University Press, 1988.

Susie, Debra Anne. *In the Way of Our Grandmothers: A Cultural View of Twentieth-Century Midwifery in Florida.* Athens: University of Georgia Press, 1988.

Susser, Ida. "Poverty and Homelessness in U.S. Cities." In *Cultural Diversity in the United States,* ed. Ida Susser and Thomas Patterson, 229–249. Malden, MA: Blackwood, 2001.

————. "Working-Class Women, Social Protest, and Changing Ideologies." In *Women and the Politics of Empowerment,* ed. Ann Bookman and Sandra Morgen, 257–272. Philadelphia: Temple University Press, 1988.

Taylor, Janelle, Linda Layne, and Danielle Wozniak, eds. *Consuming Motherhood.* New Brunswick, NJ: Rutgers University Press, 2004.

Taylor, Verta. "Social Movement Continuity: The Women's Movement in Abeyance." *American Sociological Review* 54, no. 5 (1989): 761–775.

Tom, Sally Austen. "The Evolution of Nurse-Midwifery: 1900–1960." *Journal of Nurse-Midwifery* 27, no. 4 (July–August 1982): 4–13.

Treichler, Paula. "Feminism, Medicine, and the Meaning of Childbirth." In *Body/Politics: Women and the Discourse of Science,* ed. Mary Jacobus, Evelyn Fox Keller, and Sally Shuttleworth, 113–138. New York: Routledge, 1990.

Trunzo, C. E. "Children: Special Deliveries." *Money Magazine* 12 (December, 1983): 205–206, 208, 211.

Underwood, Felix. "Development of Midwifery in Mississippi." *Southern Medical Journal* 19 (1926): 683–685.

U.S. Census Bureau. "Income and Poverty in 1999, Virginia, by County," 2000. Available at www.factfinder.census.gov, accessed December 5, 2007.

———. "Poverty Thresholds in 1999 by Size of Family and Number of Related Children under 18 Years Old," 2000. Available at www.factfinder.census.gov, accessed December 5, 2007.

United Nations General Assembly. "Universal Declaration of Human Rights," adopted by General Assembly Resolution 217 A (III), December 10, 1948.

van Blarcom, Carolyn Conant. "Rat Pie among the Black Midwives of the South." *Harper's Monthly Magazine* (February 1930): 322–332.

van Olphen-Fehr, Juliana. *Diary of a Midwife: The Power of Positive Childbearing.* Westport, CT: Bergin and Garvey, 1998.

Virginia Chapter of the American College of Nurse Midwives. "About the VA Chapter." Available at www.vamidwife.org/aboutus.html, accessed July 3, 2008; last updated April 12, 2006.

Virginia Friends of Midwives. "Virginia Friends of Midwives." Available at www.vfom .org, accessed July 6, 2003; last updated June 23, 2003.

Virginia State Board of Health. "Midwife Instruction: A Series of Lectures." Prepared for Nurses. Richmond: Virginia Board of Health, 1924.

Visweswaran, Kamala. *Fictions of Feminist Ethnography.* Minneapolis: University of Minnesota Press, 1994.

———. "Histories of Feminist Ethnography." *Annual Review of Anthropology* 26 (1997): 591–621.

Voices for Healthcare Rights Fund. "Alternative Healthcare Practitioners: Endangered Species." Fund-raising brochure. Toano, VA: Voices for Healthcare Rights Fund, 1999.

———. "Stafford Case against Midwives Unravels amidst New Questions." Press release, May 2, 2000.

Wagner, Marsden. "A Modern-Day Witch Hunt in Virginia: One Mother's Death Should Not Derail Midwife Legislation." *Roanoke Times,* February 3, 1999, A13.

Ward, Jule DeJager. *La Leche League: At the Crossroads of Medicine, Feminism, and Religion.* Chapel Hill: University of North Carolina Press, 2000.

Warner, Mark R. "Statement of Governor Mark R. Warner on the 75th Anniversary of the *Buck vs. Bell* Decision," May 2, 2002. Available at www.hsc.virginia.edu/ medicine/inter-dis/bio-ethics/warner%20apology.PDF, accessed July 17, 2003.

Warshaw, R. "The American Way of Birth: High Tech Hospitals, Birthing Centers, or No Options at All." *Ms. Magazine* 13 (September 1984): 45–50, 130.

Waterston, Alisse, and Maria Vesperi, eds. *Anthropology off the Shelf: Anthropologists on Writing.* New York: Blackwell, 2009.

Weisman, Carol S. *Women's Health Care: Activist Traditions and Institutional Change.* Baltimore, MD: Johns Hopkins University Press, 1998.

Wertz, Richard W., and Dorothy C. Wertz. *Lying-In.* New York: Free Press, 1979.

Wessel, Helen S. *Natural Childbirth and the Christian Family.* New York: Harper and Row, 1963.

Whiteford, Linda M. "Political Economy, Gender, and the Social Production of Health and Illness." In *Gender and Health: An International Perspective*, ed. Carolyn F. Sargent and Caroline B. Brettell, 242–259. Upper Saddle River, NJ: Prentice Hall, 1996.

Williams, Brett. "Babies and Banks: The 'Reproductive Underclass' and the Raced, Gendered Masking of Debt." In *Race*, ed. Steven Gregory and Roger Sanjek, 348–365. New Brunswick, NJ: Rutgers University Press, 1996.

Index

Abortion and contraception: and choice, 2, 4; compulsory, 118; debates over, 7, 29–30, 85–86, 155–156n28; and eugenics, 31, 145; and herbal preparations, 155n25; legalization of abortion, 39; and midwives, 156n31; and natural childbirth movement, 49; as rights, 119–120; underground, 159n109

Abortion and the Politics of Motherhood, 120

Abu-Lughod, Lila, x, 13–14

Activism, ix–xiv, 17–18, 22, 161n34; and natural childbirth movement, 50; and midwifery, 55, 75–78; and neoliberalism, 132–138; and women's rights, 118. *See also* Consumer activism; Political activism; Reproductive rights activism

Activist mothering, 97

Activist Scholarship, 13–17

African American Midwifery in the South, 63

African American midwives, 33, 51, 57–58, 66, 78, 158nn94, 95, 164–165n122; and birth registration, 63; elimination of, 7, 22, 25, 38, 61, 62–67, 78; and Sheppard-Towner Maternal and Infancy Protection Act, 37–38; training of, 68–69. *See also* Granny midwives

African Americans: and abortion, 4; and access to healthcare, 34, 87; and birth control, 31–32; and government, 106; and hospital births, 166n23; and medical progress, 38; and midwives, 59, 61; and mortality rates, 65; and prenatal care, 87; and the Sheppard-Towner Maternal and Infancy Protection Act, 7; and sterilization, 31–32, 36

American Academy of Pediatrics, 171n19

American Birth Control League, 30

American College of Home Obstetrics (ACHO), 44

American College of Nurse-Midwives (ACNM), 67, 69, 77–78, 171n15

American College of Obstetricians and Gynecologists (ACOG), 139, 171n19

American Indian midwives, 63

American Indians, 63, 106, 165n9

American Medical Association, 28, 30, 34, 35, 38, 139–140

American Society for Psychoprophylaxis in Obstetrics (ASPO), 42

Anesthesia, 42, 157nn53, 67, 163n90

Anthropology, 17–18

Arms, Suzanne, 52

Association for Childbirth at Home International (ACHI), 44

Attachment parenting, 110

Baer, Hans, 28

Bailis, Alice, 70

Baxandall, Rosalyn, 26, 27
Bearing Meaning, 43
Beggars and Choosers, 120
Bentheim, Steven, 88–90
Big Push for Midwives, 1, 12, 40, 55, 139
Biggs, Lesley, 13, 41
Bing, Elizabeth, 42
Biomedicine, 27, 28. *See also* Medicine
Birth centers, 69, 70
Birth in Four Cultures, 43
Birth registration, 63
BirthCare and Women's Health, 69, 70
Black, Dick, 142
Blessed Events, 46, 61
Block, Jennifer, 48, 54, 56, 74
Bobel, Chris, 53, 110, 112
Borst, Charlotte, 59
Bourgeault, Ivy Lynn, ix, 125
Breastfeeding, 42, 49, 83, 111
Breckinridge, Mary, 150n7
Breech birth, 128
A Brief History of Neoliberalism, 10
Brown, Michael, 103
Buck v. Bell, 118, 176n11
Buck, Carrie, 118

Cahn, Naomi, 53
Cahours, Carol, 71
Caillagh, Cynthia, 72–75, 168n72
Canada, ix, 11, 28, 133, 143, 151n33, 163n82
Carnegie Foundation, 28
Carter, Patricia Cloyd, 46
Cassidy, Tina, 48
Certified midwives (CMs), 150n1, 171n15
Certified nurse-midwives (CNMs), 1, 68–69,
    82, 96, 154n80; and certified professional
    midwives (CPMs), 78; demand for access
    to, 69; and homebirth, 70, 77, 76; and
    hospital births, 58–59; physician
    supervision of, x, 2, 12, 13, 45, 55, 68–69,
    78, 140–141; support for direct-entry
    midwives (DEMs), 83; urbanization of,
    169n84; and white mothers, 59; working
    outside their profession, 69
Certified professional midwives (CPMs), 72, 78,
    150n1; and controlled substances, 96; and
    labor complications, 85; legal access to, 1;
    licensing of, x, 13, 77–78, 81, 82, 84–86,
    94–95, 173n41; physician supervision of,
    95–96; and prescriptive authority, 140–141;
    training, 90
Cesarean sections, 53, 56, 74, 85, 127
Chafe, William, 34

Chicago Maternity Center, 45
Child abuse, 88, 90
Child custody, 109
Childbirth: and choice, 51; cultural
    differences, 43; deaths, 33–34; differing
    experiences in, 41, 59; literature, 42,
    50–51; and pain, 21, 32–33, 42, 43, 48, 65,
    157nn53, 67, 163n90; and socioeconomic
    status, 57, 59, 65–66. *See also* Homebirth;
    Hospital births; Medicalized childbirth;
    Natural childbirth; "Primitive childbirth"
Childbirth reform, 22, 43–44, 44–45, 46, 57
Childbirth services, 33; access to, 57; and
    consumers, 56–57; and socioeconomic
    status, 32–33
Childbirth Wisdom, 52
Childbirth without Fear, 42
Children's Bureau, 34, 37–38, 65
Choice: and abortion and contraception, 2,
    119; "bad" and "good", 90, 120; and
    childbirth, 1–2, 4–5, 51, 56–57; and
    childbirth reform, 43, 57, 111; and
    consumer identity, 4–5, 6, 11, 105; and
    consumer rights, 121; and feminism, 8, 48,
    137; and homebirth, 21, 22, 23, 48, 85–86,
    88–89, 91–94, 101–102; language of, 2, 3,
    126; and midwifery, 5, 21–22, 58, 115–116,
    121–132; and natural childbirth, 54; and
    reproductive health services, 118; and
    socioeconomic status, 3, 125–132
Citizens, 115, 177n23
Citizens for Midwifery (CfM), 55–56
Citizens' rights, 11, 116–117, 120–121,
    144–145
Citizenship, 117
Civil Rights Act of 1964, 35, 67, 117–118,
    166n23
Civil rights movement, 4, 24, 38, 118, 120
Civil War, 27
Cochran, Steve, 76
Code of Virginia, 67–68
Commonwealth Midwives Alliance (CMA),
    77
Constitution of the United States, 121, 123,
    124, 140; Equal Protection Clause, 120;
    Nineteenth Amendment, 34, 117
Consumer education, 128–129
Consumer groups, 143
Consumer movement, 42, 177n23
Consumer rights, 9–11, 40–60, 120–121,
    177n23; and choice, 4–5, 56, 56–57, 121,
    121–132; for low income women, 16; and
    midwifery care, 2–3, 115–116, 132,

143–144; and reproductive rights, 3, 21, 23; rhetoric of, 146–147; and socioeconomic status, 115, 146

Consuming Motherhood, 5

Contraception. *See* Abortion and contraception

Cosminsky, Sheila, 57

Cosslett, Tess, 51, 52

Counterculture movement, 46–47

Cruikshank, Barbara, 121

Davis-Floyd, Robbie, 1, 5, 25, 57, 80, 82, 144

De Vries, Raymond, 45–46, 49, 55, 144

DeLee, Joseph B., 45, 164–165n122

Democratic Party, 9

Dick-Read, Grantley, 42, 44, 46

Direct-entry midwives (DEMs): certification of, 1; decriminalization of, 74, 74, 75, 77, 128–129; definition of, 150n1; legal status of, 2, 12–13, 55, 70, 76–78, 170–171n14; licensing of, 57, 81–82, 83, 88, 94, 128, 168n67; prohibition against, 123; regulation of, 173n41; underground, 154n80; and white mothers, 59

Doulas, 56

Ebbin, Adam, 142

Edwards, Margot, 38, 49

Ehrenreich, Barbara, 27, 28

Eisenstadt v. Baird, 120

Engaged Observer, 15

English, Deirdre, 27, 28

Eugenics movement, 4, 29, 31, 32, 33, 36, 63, 65, 145, 165n7; and Germany, 156n45

Evans, Sara, 117

The Experience of Childbirth, 42

Families for Natural Living (FNL), 76

The Farm, 47

Farm Midwifery Center, 47

Feminism: and choice, 4, 126; and consumer identity, 136–137; and homebirth, 48; and natural childbirth, 48–49, 49–50; and politics, 99; and reproductive rights, 8

Feminist ethnography, ix–xi, x, 13–17

Fertility control, 7, 21, 24, 25, 29–32, 241

Fetal rights, 85–86, 169n76

Fiedler, Deborah Cordero, 1

Fierro, Marcella, 168n67

Finkbine, Sherri, 119

Flexner Report, 27–28

Flexner, Abraham, 28

Foucault, Michel, 10, 80

Fraser, Gertrude, 8, 24, 25, 33, 37, 38, 58, 59, 62, 63, 65

Fredericksburg Area Consumers of Homebirth and Midwifery Care, 76

The Free Lance-Star, 74

Frontier Nursing School, 150n7

Gaskin, Ina May, 46–47

Genocide, 32

Ginsburg, Faye, 3, 30

Goldsmith, Judith, 52

Goodman, Debbie, 75

Gordon, Linda, 26, 27, 31

Government regulation: of abortion and contraception, 29; of childbirth, 22, 74, 83; of direct-entry midwives (DEMs), 55, 76–77; and homebirth, 50; of midwives, 34, 66–67, 79, 128–129; and the poor, 35; of women's bodies, 85

Government surveillance, 7, 10, 24, 37, 63, 65, 80, 83, 164n113, 172n22

Granny midwives, 36, 51, 57–58, 62, 66, 70, 158n94

Granny Midwives and Black Women Writers, 36

Grassroots organizing and organizations, 19, 22, 103–105, 112, 115, 141–142, 146; and direct-entry midwives (DEMs), 2; and market-based arguments, 136; and socioeconomic status, 132–135

Grassroots Warriors, 97, 98

Greenspun, Peter, 73

Grewal, Inderpal, 118

Griswold v. Connecticut, 119

Hale, Charles, 15

Hale, Edwin M., 155n28

Haley, James Jr., 74

Halfmoon, Hygeia, 54

Hamblet, Ellen, 69, 91–94, 123

Haraway, Donna, x–xi

Harrison, Faye, 14

Harrisonburg Advocates for the Midwifery Model of Care (HAMMOC), 76

Harvey, David, 10

Haw, Elizabeth, 72–75

Health insurance. *See* Insurance: health

Healthcare reform, 34

Herbalists, 27

Hippies. *See* Counterculture movement

Holmes, Linda Janet, 38

Holmes, Oliver Wendell, 118

Homebirth: as alternative to hospital birth, 44; as challenge to American values, 173n36; as child abuse, 88, 90; and choice, 91–94; and Constitution of the United States, 124; and criminal prosecutions of midwives, 72–75; and deaths, 168n67; and demographic data, 164n113; feminist support of, 48; interest in, 70; legality of, 67, 89; and midwifery, 61; opposition to, 61, 65–66, 139–140; and pathological motherhood, 88–90; as a political act, 50, 110–114; and poverty, 133; and race, 58; and religion, 86, 86; as a reproductive right, 1–23; and risk, 83, 84–85, 87, 90, 171n19, 173n28; and socioeconomic status, 11, 35, 109; support for, 55–60, 143; unassisted, 50, 54, 109, 175n28; underground midwife attended, 109–110

Homebirth mothers: activism among, 75–78; alliance of, 40; and American values, 87; as "bad" mothers, 79, 83, 85, 88, 90, 95, 98; choices of, 22, 86–87, 105; as consumers, 6, 11, 80, 96, 97, 115–116, 123, 125, 134, 143, 146; demographics of, 140; disrespect of, 98, 102–103, 109; diversity of, 19, 99–100, 154n73; as educated consumers, 91–94; fear of repercussions from the state, 97–98, 108, 112, 129–130, 132, 164n113; and healthcare system, 100; and legislative hearings, 23, 80–81, 100–103; as lobbyists for midwives, 79–80; and midwives, 82–83, 99, 121–122, 125, 135, 137, 141; and organizing, 22, 23; and political activism, 97–98, 103–105; political and religious diversity of, 12, 116, 125, 126, 154n73; political experiences of, 105–110; and politics, 98–100; and reproductive rights, 1–23; and socioeconomic status, 12, 41, 70–71; and the state, 101; terminology for, 4–6, 124–125, 134–135; vilification of, 83–84

Homebirth movement, 12, 40, 44, 45, 47, 55, 71; and socioeconomic status, 19

Homebirth organizations, 44

Homeopathic practitioners, 27

Hospital births, 53–54, 94–95, 139; and bad experiences, 92; and disrespect, 98, 109; and doulas, 56; and immigrants, 59; and midwives, 58–59; and pain, 32, 65; procedures in, 160n23; as rape, 101–102; reform, 43–44; and respectable motherhood, 80; and segregation, 166n23;

and socioeconomic status, 35, 44–45, 58–59, 65–66; and twilight sleep, 157n67

Howard University, 28

Howell, Janet, 94

Hughes, Martha, 72

Human rights, 118, 120, 176n7

Hyatt, Susan, 89

Immaculate Deception, 52

Immigrant midwives, 29, 33, 164–165n122; elimination of, 7, 25; and Sheppard-Towner Maternal and Infancy Protection Act, 37

Immigrants, 36, 59, 61

In Labor, 40, 54

Incapacitated adult, neglect of, 73, 74, 75

Infant healthcare reform. *See* Maternal and infant healthcare reform

Informed Homebirth, 44

Insurance: health, 55, 57, 130, 133, 140, 144–145; malpractice, 87

International Childbirth Education Association (ICEA), 42

Jackson, Marsha, 70

Jane Collective, 159n109

Jenkins, Susan, 139–140

Jim Crow laws, 36

Jordan, Brigitte, 43, 85

Kahn, Robbie Pfeufer, 42, 43

Karmel, Marjorie, 42

Kessler-Harris, Alice, 121

Kingfisher, Catherine, 11

Kitzinger, Sheila, 42, 43

Klassen, Pamela, 3, 6, 42, 46, 56, 61, 86

Krauss, Celene, 106

La Leche League (LLL), 42, 49

Labor Pains, 44

Ladd-Taylor, Molly, 36, 37

Lamaze method, 42, 44

Lamaze, Ferdinand, 42

Laughlin, Harry, 156n45

Lay health practitioners, 26, 27

Lay midwives, 45–46, 58, 71, 167n39; criminalization of, 22, 67–70; elimination of, 37; replacement with nurse midwives, 51, 68

Leavitt, Judith Walzer, 32, 45

Lee, Valerie, 36

Legislative hearings, 79, 86–87, 88–90, 173n28; children at, 80–82, 106–107, 170n7; homebirth mother's testimony at,

91–94; and legislators, 84–85, 100–101; and midwife supporters, 22; midwife supporters' testimony at, 90–91; and race, 73
LeHew, Willette, 88
Licensed midwives (LMs), 150n1
Listservs, 12, 77; and privacy, 153–154n71
Luker, Kristen, 119, 120
Lying-In, 35

Macari, Marcie, 52–53
MacDonald, Margaret, ix, 5, 51, 54, 125
Making Midwives Legal, 45–46
Markets, 9–10, 120–121, 129, 132
Maskovsky, Jeff, 11
Maternal and infant healthcare reform, 33–39, 35–37
Maternity Center (Bethesda, MD), 70
Mathews, Holly, 37, 57–58
Matthews, Jean, 30
Mead, Margaret, 43, 160n17
Medicaid, 57, 67, 134, 140, 141
Medical associations, 78
Medical College of Virginia Hospital (MCV), 166n23
Medical lobby, ix, 35, 38, 102–103, 172n24
Medical malpractice liability, 57
Medical schools, 27–28
Medical Society of Virginia (MSV), 82, 83
Medicalized childbirth, 53–54, 66, 84–86; alternatives to, 79; critiques of, 3, 25, 39, 46; differing experiences with, 25, 59–60; as a monopoly, 124; and natural childbirth, 115; patriarchal origins of, 50; as rape, 101–102; resistance to, 26, 38; and respectable motherhood, 86–87; and risk, 87; superiority of, 22
Medicine, 41, 172n22. *See also* Biomedicine
Meharry Medical College, 28
Michie, Helena, 53
Midwife legislation, 79–96, 133, 173n41; and access, 57; in Arizona, 55; bipartisan support for, 142; and certified professional midwives, 77, 78, 140; and children, 106–107; and consumer rights, 115, 116, 123; in Costa Rica, 166n16; debates over, 22; decriminalization, 74; defeat of, 83; and direct-entry midwives (DEMs), 12, 75; in Florida, 55, 57, 142; and homebirth mothers, 22; in Mississippi, 55; and neoliberalism, 21; and non-nurse midwives, 67–68; in North Carolina, 57–58; successes, 94–96

Midwifery care: access to, 1–3, 8, 12–13, 18, 22, 40, 50, 55, 57, 58, 77, 102, 116, 123, 141, 144; and African Americans, 59; and choice, 58; consumers of, 121–132; decriminalization of, 82; and financial issues, 130–132; and homebirth, 61; impact of medicine on, 41; market for, 137; medical opposition to, 78; and natural childbirth, 51; and race, 58; rediscovery of, 70–75; restrictions on, 55; and socioeconomic status, 66, 116; support for, 55–60, 59–60; and white women, 8, 19, 21, 33, 35, 37, 51, 55, 57–59, 66, 70, 73, 110, 134
Midwifery movement, x–xi, 5, 12, 23, 54, 116, 122, 124, 125, 133–135, 137; and consumer activism, 21, 40–60; histories of, 41
Midwifery Options for Mothers (MOM), 76
Midwifery permits, 64, 67, 68, 168n71, 173n41
Midwifery support organizations, 60, 76–78
Midwifery supporters, 17, 81, 96; and childbirth experiences, 145; community based, 110; as consumers, 56, 121–123; diversity of, x–xi, 12, 143; experiences in the legislature, 101–102; fear of repercussions from the state, 106; homebirth mothers, 79–80, 99; language of, 2, 145; and male legislators, 100–103; and midwife protection, 153–154n71; and midwifery legislation, 82, 140; and political activism, 97–98, 103–105; political and religious diversity of, xiii, 6, 12, 19, 60, 115, 137, 143; political experiences, 105–110; and race, 21; and socioeconomic status, 11, 19–21, 61, 97–98, 105–110, 110–114, 132–135, 134; stereotypes of, 22; strategies of, 13, 21; as volunteers, 103
Midwifery Task Force of Ontario (MTFO), 143
Midwives: and abortion, 29, 156n31; activism for, 75–78; campaigns against, 65–66; as commodities, 5–6; and community, 130–131; community based, 7; and compensation, 68, 71–72, 167n35; and consumers, 54, 125; criminal prosecutions of, 72–74, 152n49; definitions of, 68, 71–72; diversity of, 70–71; in the early 1900s, 62–67; education of, 62–63; elderly, 64–65; elimination of, 38; fear of repercussions from the state, 78; feminist support of, 48; and homebirth mother terminology, 124–125; and homebirth mothers, 125, 135; legalization of, 22;

Midwives: and abortion (*cont.*)
  licensing of, 25, 63–64, 76–77, 79, 141; and
    manslaughter charges, 72; morality of, 64;
    obligations to the state, 64; opposition to,
    37, 61; with permits, 68; and physicians,
    66–67; and the poor, 36–37; practicing
    without a license, 72–75, 152n49, 168n71;
    and racial stereotypes, 59; rules for, 168.71;
    supervision of, 62–63; support for, 92, 143;
    training of, 64, 83; and Twilight Sleep,
    157n67; unlicensed, xii, 71–72; versatility
    of, xiv. *See also* African American midwives;
    American Indian midwives; Certified
    nurse-midwives; Certified professional
    midwives; Direct-entry midwives; Granny
    midwives; Immigrant midwives; Lay
    midwives; Underground midwives
Midwives Alliance of North America
    (MANA), x, 2, 146
Midwives and Mothers in Action Campaign
    (MAMA), 1, 12, 40, 55–56
Midwives Model of Care, 56
Miller, Linda, 57
Milton, Gladys, 57
Milton, Maria, 57
Mohanty, Chandra Talpade, 115
Montagu, Ashley, 43
Morgen, Sandra, 8, 98
Mortality rates, 33, 38, 41, 63, 65
Motherhood, 30; and choice, 53; and
    consumption, 5; definitions of, 41; and
    homebirth, 88–90; obligatory, 48
Mothers: activist, 98–99; drug addicted, 89;
    and "good" decisions, 83; respectable, 6,
    79–80, 83, 86–87, 90–91, 96, 97. *See also*
    Homebirth mothers
Mothers United for Midwifery (MUM), 76
My Bag Was Always Packed, 67

Nader, Ralph, 120
Naples, Nancy, 97, 98
National Association of Parents and
    Professionals for Safe Alternatives in
    Childbirth (NAPSAC), 44, 49
National Black Women's Health Project, 31
National Organization for Women (NOW), 48
Native Americans. *See* American Indians
Natural childbirth, 25, 145, 162–163n79; and
    choice, 53–54; definitions of, 54; failure to
    achieve, 53; feminist support of, 48; in the
    hospital, 160n17; instructional manuals, 50;
    methods, 42; and pain, 53; reassessment of,
    51–53; and socioeconomic status, 33

Natural childbirth movement, ix, 3, 4, 12, 39,
    41–46, 55, 120, 145; and abortion, 49; and
    activism, 50; and consumer identification,
    115; as a consumer movement, 42;
    similarities within, 47–48; diversity in, 40,
    46–50, 56; and feminism, 48, 49–50; and
    midwives, 45–46; political and religious
    diversity in, 40, 46–50, 56; and
    socioeconomic status, 8, 21–22, 25, 50–54
"Natural mothering", 112
Nelson, Margaret, 51, 53
Neoliberalism, 9–11, 152nn36, 38, 177n23;
    and activism, 132–138; and citizens' rights,
    120–121; and consumer rights, 23,
    144–145, 146–147; and midwife legislation,
    21; and midwifery supporters, 122; and
    policy shifts, 12; and reproductive rights,
    115
Nestel, Sheryl, 11, 133
Newby, Stacy, 71
Nineteenth Amendment. *See* Constitution of
    the United States: Nineteenth Amendment
No Time for Fear, 42
Norman, Bari Meltzer, 85–86
North American Registry of Midwives, 82, 96
Nurse-midwives, 67, 150n7. *See also* Certified
    nurse-midwives (CNMs)

OB/GYN doctors. *See* Physicians
Obstetrics, 25, 43, 45
Oleson, Eric, 74
Online social networking groups, 12
Ontario Midwifery Consumer Network
    (OMCN), 143
Ordover, Nancy, 118–119
Osbourne, Susan, 72

Painless Childbirth, 42
The Paradox of Natural Mothering, 110
Parental rights, 83, 88–89
Parker, Jennifer, 58–59
Partridge, John, 84–85, 87
Patel, Raj, 144–145
Peninsula Families for Natural Birth and
    Health Care (PenFam), 76
Petchesky, Rosalind, 29–30
Peters, Claire, 74, 168n72
Peters, Daren, 73
Peters, Julia, 72–75, 168n72
Peterson, Anne, 86–87, 92
Physicians, 27, 28, 37, 87. *See also* Certified
    nurse-midwives: physician supervision of;
    Midwives: and Physicians

Pigg, Stacey Leigh, 57
Planned Parenthood, 30, 31
Plecker, Walter, 62–63, 165n9
Policies, healthcare. *See* Healthcare policies
Political activism, 97–100, 118; definitions of, 103–105; and fear of repercussions from the state, 108, 110
Popular health movement, 7, 21, 26–29, 145; success of, 27
Population control, 31
Potter, Brynne, 77, 140, 151n9
Preceptors, 82
Pregnancy and Power, 79
"Primitive childbirth", 41, 51–53, 54, 162–163n79
Prown, Katherine, 151n9, 163n96
Pushed!, 74

Racial Integrity Acts, 63, 165n9
Racism, 4, 8, 106, 164–165n122. *See also* African American midwives: elimination of; Childbirth: and socioeconomic status; Childbirth services: and socioeconomic status; Hospital births: and socioeconomic status; Immigrant midwives: elimination of; Natural childbirth: and socioeconomic status; Natural childbirth movement: and socioeconomic status; Reproductive healthcare services: and socioeconomic status; Reproductive rights: and socioeconomic status; Women's rights: and socioeconomic inequalities
Rakowitz, Elly, 42
Rapp, Rayna, 3, 127
Reclaiming Birth, 38, 49
Reid, Margaret, 47
Religion, 86
Reproductive healthcare policies, 2, 7, 9–10
Reproductive healthcare reform, 3, 7, 26–29, 35, 137. *See also* Maternal and infant healthcare reform
Reproductive healthcare services: access to, 38–39; and incarcerated women, 10; consumption of, 6; inequities in, 11, 24–25, 36–37; medical management of, 83; and socioeconomic status, 7–8, 25
Reproductive justice, 4, 6
Reproductive rights, 49; activism, ix; and citizenship, 119; and consumer identity, 136–137; as consumer rights, 2, 3–7, 9–11, 115; and eugenics, 145; as human rights, 118, 120; language of, 3, 16; and midwifery care, 2–3; and neoliberalism, 9, 137–138;

and religion, 86, 86; and reproductive choices, 135; and socioeconomic status, 8, 117, 144, 146, 146–147; as women's rights, 119–120. *See also* Choice
Reproductive rights movement, 1–23; and feminism, 48; history of, 7–8, 21, 24–39, 146; and midwifery supporters, 96; and neoliberalism, 23
Republican Party, 9
Reverby, Susan, 26, 27
Richmond Families for Birthing Alternatives (RFBA), 76
Right to life, 85, 118, 120
Right to privacy, 119–120, 140
Rights, 116–121, 123–124. *See also* Citizens' rights; Consumer rights; Fetal rights; Human rights; Parental rights; Reproductive rights; Voting rights; Women's rights
The Roanoke Times, 75
Roberson, Mildred, 67
Roe v. Wade, 39, 120
Romalis, Shelley, 53
Ross, Loretta, 31
Roth, Rachel, 74
Rothman, Barbara Katz, 5, 40, 44, 54, 85–86
Ruzek, Sheryl Burt, 47–48, 129, 145–146

Sandelowski, Margarete, 32, 43, 49
Sanford, Victoria, 15
Sanger, Margaret, 30
Sawicki, Jana, 53
She Births, 52–53
Sheppard-Towner Maternal and Infancy Protection Act, 7, 21, 34–35, 36–38, 38, 65, 117, 173n36
Shryock, Richard, 34
Simonds, Wendy, 85–86
Simple living, 19, 110
Skinner v. Oklahoma, 118
Skinner, Jack T., 119
Skocpol, Theda, 34
Smith, Claudine Curry, 66
Smith, Margaret Charles, 38
Social reform movements, 26–27
Solinger, Rickie, 3, 4, 29, 31, 41, 79, 118, 120, 135, 136
Spiritual Midwifery, 47
St. Phillips Hospital, 166n23
Stacey, Judith, 13–14
Stanton, Elizabeth Cady, 30
Sterilization, 4, 29, 31, 36, 65, 118–119, 156n45, 165nn7, 9

Stratified reproduction, 3, 11, 21, 24, 25, 117, 127, 146
Sullivan, Deborah, 44
Supreme Court of the United States, 118, 119, 120
Susie, Debra, 50–51, 67

Thank You, Dr. Lamaze, 42
Tom, Sally Austen, 35
Treichler, Paula, 48
Twilight Sleep, 32–33, 157n67

Underground midwives, 17, 19, 72, 76, 109–110
Underwood, Felix, 164–165n122
United Nations Charter, 118

VABirthPAC, 141–142
van Olphen-Fehr, Juliana, 70–71
Virginia, xi–xii, 2, 12–13, 23, 55
Virginia Birthing Freedom (VBF), 76, 91
Virginia Board of Medicine, 69
Virginia Bureau of Vital Statistics, 62, 63
Virginia Chapter of the American College of Nurse-Midwives (VA-ACNM), 77–78
Virginia Chapter of the American College of Obstetricians and Gynecologists (VA-ACOG), 82, 83, 84, 88, 93, 171n19, 173n28
Virginia Department of Health (VDH), 66–67, 68, 76, 76, 82, 86
Virginia Department of Health Professionals (VDHP), 76, 82, 142
Virginia Friends of Midwives (VFOM), x
Virginia General Assembly, 66, 67–68, 74, 75, 76, 80–83, 102–103
Virginia legislative committees: Governor's Work Group on Rural Obstetrical Care, x, 137, 179n3; Health, Welfare, and Institutions Committee (HWI), 83, 84, 86, 88, 91; Joint Commission on Health Care (JCHC), 12, 69, 76, 77, 81–82, 170–171n14; Maternal and Child Health Council, 76; Task Force on the Study of Obstetric Access and Certified Nurse-Midwives, 68, 69
Virginia Medical Society (VMS), 93
Virginia Midwifery Coalition (VMC), 77, 121–122
Virginia Obstetrical and Gynecological Society (VA OB/GYN), 82, 83, 84, 88
Virginia Sterilization Act of 1924, 165n9
Voices for Healthcare Rights Fund (Voices), 75, 76
Voting rights, 34, 117

Wagner, Marsden, 75
Waldorf, Mary, 38, 49
Weisman, Carol, 29
Weitz, Rose, 44
Wertz, Dorothy, 33, 35, 36
Wertz, Richard, 33, 35, 36
Wessel, Helen, 46
Willis, Sherry, 71
Wilson, Adella Scott, 167n39
Wisconsin, 156n31
Woman's Body, Woman's Right, 31
Women, 28, 74. *See also* Homebirth mothers; Mothers
Women as Mothers, 43
Women Writing Childbirth, 51
Women's bodies, control over, 24, 29, 30, 31, 38, 79, 80, 85, 126, 135, 172n22
Women's health movement, 3, 8, 118
Women's lobby, 38
Women's rights, 30, 34–35, 115; as human rights, 176n7; and motherhood, 48; and socioeconomic inequalities, 117–118
Women's rights movement, 26–27, 48, 161n34
World Health Organization, 75
World War I, 35